IMPROVING THE QUALITY OF LIFE: RECOMMENDATIONS FOR PEOPLE WITH AND WITHOUT DISABILITIES

Library of Congress Cataloging-in-Publication Data

A C.I.P. Catalogue record for this book is available from the Library of Congress.

ISBN 0-7923-3234-2

Published by Kluwer Academic Publishers,
P.O. Box 17, 3300 AA Dordrecht, The Netherlands.

Kluwer Academic Publishers incorporates
the publishing programmes of
D. Reidel, Martinus Nijhoff, Dr W. Junk and MTP Press.

Sold and distributed in the U.S.A. and Canada
by Kluwer Academic Publishers,
101 Philip Drive, Norwell, MA 02061, U.S.A.

In all other countries, sold and distributed
by Kluwer Academic Publishers Group,
P.O. Box 322, 3300 AH Dordrecht, The Netherlands.

Printed on acid-free paper

Printed in the Netherlands

IMPROVING THE QUALITY OF LIFE

Recommendations for People with and without Disabilities

Edited by

DAVID M. ROMNEY
University of Calgary, Alberta, Canada

ROY I. BROWN
Flinders University, Adelaide, South Australia

and

PREM S. FRY
University of Victoria, British Columbia, Canada

Reprinted from Social Indicators Research 33 (1–3), 1994

KLUWER ACADEMIC PUBLISHERS
DORDRECHT / BOSTON / LONDON

TABLE OF CONTENTS

GUEST EDITORIAL

This collection of papers is based primarily on a colloquium series on *Improving the Quality of Life in Normal and Disabled Populations* that was held at the University of Calgary during the Fall of 1991 as part of the celebration in honour of the University's 25th Anniversary. However, this publication goes well beyond the original proceedings in terms of the depth and scope of reviews of the literature, with the addition of papers from two authors who did not participate in the colloquium series and a concluding paper written by the editors. Efforts have been made to provide recommendations for research and practice along with suggestions for future development in the field of quality of life.

The idea to have a colloquium series on improving quality of life occurred when we realized that although much had been written about the topic, most had to do with its conceptualization and measurement, and very little was concerned with its improvement. We were struck by the urgent need for practical recommendations based on empirical research findings and theory that could help individuals or services make a difference to quality of life. We were also impressed by the fact that there were distinct populations ranging from young people with developmental disabilities to people who are old and frail, and from those with chronic mental disorders (e.g., schizophrenia) to those with chronic physical illnesses (e.g., AIDS) who all had challenges relating to quality of life resulting from their disabilities. To some considerable degree the literature on these populations was compartmentalized. This anomaly was brought home on one occasion when a colleague working in the field of chronic physical illness surprised another who was working in the field of developmental disabilities by asking him if there had been much work done on the topic of quality of life in that population!

It was then that we formed a small group within the University to plan and organize a series of workshops to be conducted by invited experts. The three of us, Roy Brown, Prem Fry and David Romney, stayed the course and, when we decided that the series would be worth publishing, continued our collaboration as co-editors. Roy Brown's area is developmental disabilities and rehabilitation. He has recently published (with Max Bayer) a scale for assessing quality of life in that population and has attempted to apply quality of life models to practical programs. Prem Fry has concentrated on life-span development and gerontology and has published widely in this field. As for David Romney, his interest in quality of life stems from the time he spent in Geneva as a Consultant to the World Health Organization preparing a proposal for assessing the quality of life of individuals considered psychotic who were living in the community.

In this anthology, what constitutes quality of life, how it can be assessed and how it can be enhanced in both normal and disabled populations is examined from both theoretical and practical perspectives. The term "disability" is used in its generic sense, as sanctioned by WHO (1980), to cover "any restriction or lack ... of ability to perform in a manner or within the range considered normal for a human being". This definition encompasses both developmental and gerontological disabilities as well as those associated with chronic physical and mental illness. A unique aspect of the present enterprise, therefore, is its broad coverage, since it deals with a gamut of different populations, all of which have special needs and problems relating to assessing and improving quality of life.

Another distinct feature of the publication is its emphasis on *ameliorating* the quality of life. While much has been written on the importance of quality of life and the ways it may be assessed, concrete and feasible suggestions for bringing about beneficial changes are rarely stated explicitly. Based upon the findings from their research and upon theoretical considerations, our contributors outline the steps that need to be taken to produce tangible improvements in the quality of life of the populations they have studied.

This publication is intended for a wide audience. It will be of particular value to academics, practitioners and students or trainees in the area of rehabilitation, but it will also prove useful to specialists in psychology, sociology, social work, health, and counselling, as well as to policy makers involved in community and social services. The volume should also be of interest to individuals themselves with disabilities, to their close relatives, and to the relevant voluntary organizations.

ACKNOWLEDGEMENTS

We are indebted to the University of Calgary for subsidizing the Quality of Life Colloquium Series with a grant from the Special Projects Fund and to all the other sponsors who so kindly made financial contributions. Within the University these include the Faculty of Education, the Faculty of Social Sciences, the Department of Psychology, and the University Counselling Services. In addition, specific colloquia were funded by Care West and the Seniors Advisory Council for Alberta, the Schizophrenia Society of Alberta (Calgary Chapter), and Calgary Training and Development Consortium.

We would also like to thank personally Dr. Alex Michalos who conducted the workshop on "Improving the Quality of Life in the Normal Population" but felt that as Editor of *Social Indicators Research* it would be inappropriate for him to contribute to this special issue. Our thanks are also due to Mr. Peter de Liefde, Acquisitions Editor for Kluwer Academic Publishing, who came to Brussels last year to the International Congress of Psychology so that we could expedite the publication of the colloquium series. Finally, we gratefully acknowledge all our contributors who endeavoured to make their papers adhere to our guidelines.

ABOUT THE CONTRIBUTORS

Roy I. Brown, Ph.D., is currently Professor of Rehabilitation Studies in the Department of Educational Psychology at the University of Calgary, and has recently been invited to take up the position of Foundation Professor of Special Education and Disability Studies at Flinders University, Australia. As a practitioner and researcher, he has published extensively, and in the past few years has written a series of articles and books on the nature of quality of life as it influences people with developmental disabilities across the lifespan. He has worked extensively with people who have disabilities and has co-directed a six-year study of the quality of life of persons with developmental disabilities. He is a founder of the multidisciplinary Rehabilitation Studies program at the University of Calgary and Founding Editor of the *Journal of Practical Approaches to Developmental Handicap.*

Donna M. Cox, Ph.D., formerly Social Science Analyst at the National Institute on Aging, National Institutes of Health, Bethesda, Maryland, is currently Project Coordinator for The Long-Term Care Project. This study, conducted jointly by faculty from the University of Maryland at Baltimore and Johns Hopkins University, examines the health and health care needs of nursing home residents and how these needs differ for those with dementia. Ms. Cox recently received her doctorate in Policy Sciences at the University of Maryland Baltimore County, Baltimore, Maryland, and holds a Masters in Applied Sociology. Her areas of interests are aging and health care. She is particularly interested in the impact of the political economy on the shape and development of health and social policies in the United States.

David R. Evans, Ph.D., C.Psych., is a professor in the Clinical Psychology Program at the University of Western Ontario. Prior to coming to Western in 1971, he was in the Department of Educational Psychology at the University of Calgary. He is the author of some 70 articles, chapters, books and tests. His current research is focused on quality of life, illness prevention and health promotion. He is President Elect of the Canadian Psychological Association, a past president of the Ontario Psychological Association, and has been the Ontario representative to the American Psychological Association Council of Representatives. He has consulted with a number of community agencies, and is at present consultant to the City of London Police.

Prem S. Fry, currently Professor of Psychology and a Research Affiliate at the Centre of Aging at the University of Victoria, was formerly Professor of Educational Psychology at the University of Calgary, between 1966 and 1993. She is a Fellow of the American Psychological Association, the Canadian Psychological Association, the British Psychological Society, the American Psychological Society, and the Gerontological Society of America. Currently she holds an appointment on the Board of Directors of the Canadian Psychological Association and the Canadian Association on Gerontology. Her present research interests include stress and coping among aging women, and mediators and moderators of quality of life among elderly persons. A former Fulbright Scholar, Woodrow Wilson Scholar, and Killam Resident Fellow, she is author of six books, two monographs, and over 120 refereed journal papers and chapters. Most of her research on aging and depression has been supported by research grants from the Social Sciences and Humanities Research Council of Canada.

Dr. Halpern is Professor of Education at the University of Oregon in Eugene, Oregon where he was worked since 1970. His major interests and endeavours have been focused in the area of secondary special education and rehabilitation programs. From 1971 through 1988, he was the director of a nationally funded Rehabilitation Research and Training Center in Mental Retardation. Since 1988, he has focused most of his research and development efforts on "transition" programs for adolescents and young adults with any type of disability. During the first part of his career, Dr. Halpern developed and published 4 standardized test batteries measuring independent living skills of adolescents with mental retardation, accompanied by functional curriculum materials. He also edited a textbook on functional assessment. During recent years, his research efforts have included follow-along studies of school leavers with disabilities and studies on the dynamics of systems change within schools and adult agency programs.

Céline Mercier pursued studies in Psychology, Anthropology and in Psycholinguistics. She received her Ph.D. in Psychology from the Université Louis Pasteur (Strasbourg). She is currently Associate Professor at the Department of Psychiatry, McGill University and Director at the Psychosocial Research Unit, Douglas Hospital Research Centre and WHO Collaborating Centre. She heads a research program on the organization and evaluation of mental health services. Her interests lie mainly in the development evaluation models (pertinence, implementation and process, effectiveness and impact) adapted to community approaches, and in the use of "quality of life" as a criterion for evaluating mental health and rehabilitation services. She has carried out the evaluation of numerous intervention programs: prevention, detoxifica-tion, rehabilitation for substance abuse; crisis centres, first-line teams and community support programs for mental health. Her current work also concerns the implementation of Quebec's mental health policy, individualized service plans, and services for Montreal's homeless. Her comparative studies on the quality of life of former psychiatric patients living in the community address urban, suburban, and rural populations, in Quebec, Belgium and France. Dr. Mercier was awarded the bursary of excellence in evaluation in 1990 from the Quebec Council for Social Research.

Marcia G. Ory, Ph.D., M.P.H., is Chief, Social Science Research on Aging, Behavioral and Social Research Program, National Institute on Aging, National Institutes of Health, Bethesda, Maryland. She holds a doctorate from Purdue University and a Masters of Public Health from Johns Hopkins University. Dr. Ory is very active in professional organisations and serves on several national task forces and advisory boards dealing with aging and health issues. Her main areas of interest include aging and health care, health and behaviour research, and gender differences in health and longevity. She has published widely on these topics.

Trevor R. Parmenter, B.A., Ph.D., F.A.C.E. joined Macquarie Univer-sity in 1974 as a foundation member of the Special Education Division of the School of Education, following a 20-year teaching career in regular and special education. His doctoral dissertation explored the relation-ship between information processing strategies and the acquisition of reading skills by people with an intellectual disability. At Macquarie University his major initiative has been the establishment of the Unit for Rehabilitation Studies (recently renamed the Unit for Community Inte-gration Studies) which has been responsible for Australia's leading dis-ability research and development programs in the areas of employment, community living, transition, and systems evaluation. Professor Par-menter is the former Editor-in-Chief of the *Australia and New Zealand Journal of Developmental Disabilities* and the *Australian Disability Review*, and presently President-elect of the International Association for the Scientific Study of Intellectual Disability.

David M. Romney, Ph.D., is Professor of Clinical Psychology at the University of Calgary in Alberta, Canada. For the past 23 years he has taught full-time, and prior to that he practiced both as a clinical and as a school psychologist. In addition, he has worked in Geneva as a consultant to the World Health Organization on the quality of life issues. His current interests include schizophrenia and causal modelling and he has recently published a book (with John Bynner) on *The Structure of Personal Characteristics* which is devoted to the latter topic.

Faculty of Education   DAVID M. ROMNEY
University of Calgary   ROY I. BROWN
Calgary, Alberta   PREM S. FRY
Canada T2N 1N4

TREVOR R. PARMENTER

QUALITY OF LIFE AS A CONCEPT AND MEASURABLE ENTITY

(Accepted 14 February, 1994)

ABSTRACT. This chapter proposes that "quality of life" (QOL) is a multidimensional concept, the measurement of which must contain objective elements of a person's life. It is further suggested that in the development of QOL measurement instruments the selection of items must be influenced significantly by the views of the population under study. Instruments to measure quality of life have been flawed owing to their inadequate conceptual bases and the attempts to utilise general measures which are often the "broad brush" to detect changes in disease specific situations. The chapter outlines conceptual approaches to quality of life and provides an analysis of a range of definitions. It provides an overview of a number of approaches to measure QOL in specific populations. Finally, it addresses some of the potential uses and abuses involved in the measurement of QOL.

> *The whole of science is nothing more than a refinement of everyday thinking.*
>
> (Albert Einstein, 1950, p. 59)

As the concept of quality of life is increasingly being used a quality assurance index of the effectiveness of medical and rehabilitation services, it is appropriate to explore in some detail just what the concept means and to examine whether it is a construct that can be measured with any precision. This chapter will provide an overview of conceptual approaches to the study of quality of life in the health and rehabilitation fields and will investigate a number of efforts that have been made to operationalize the construct. Various approaches to measurement will be examined, highlighting some of the hazards involved. Specific examples of the used of scales to evaluate the effectiveness of interventions

Social Indicators Research **33:** 9–46, 1994.
© 1994 *Kluwer Academic Publishers. Printed in the Netherlands.*

in a number of disease areas will be given. A concluding section will address a number of practical and philosophical issues concerning the use of QOL scales.

A. CONCEPTUAL APPROACHES

While the use of the term"quality of life" as a scientific concept is relatively recent, it has been used colloquially in the fields of medicine and health for some time. Engel's (1978, 1980) development of a biopsychosocial model of medicine possibly heralded the emergence of the scientific application of psychosocial concepts in medicine. Applying systems theory as a framework for his formulation, Engel suggested that medicine could become a more "scientific" enterprise by the inclusion of psychosocial information in the development of medical concepts, in research and in patient care, especially when compared with the more narrow biomedical or the "nonscientific" "holistic" models. Engel's work gave a strong impetus for the broader biopsychosocial model to be incorporated into medical training and has led to medical research embracing the quality of life concept as a legitimate avenue of study.

Definitions of quality of life have ranged from unidimensional to multidimensional approaches. In the range of approaches there are some commonalities, but some quite distinct differences, particularly in terms of comprehensiveness, levels of specificity and theoretical rigour. For instance, Levine and Croog (1984) have noted that a single variable of human behaviour, such as employment, general happiness, or sexual functioning, has been used as an *ad hoc* indicator of quality of life by medical researchers. Van Dam (1986) took a somewhat similar view in suggesting that there is no clearly accepted definition of quality of life as it may refer to a variety of issues such as physical and psychological complaints, feelings of well being, sexual functioning and daily activities.

On the other hand Wegner *et al.* (1984) have proposed a more detailed three-dimensional definition (functional capacity, perceptions and symptoms) that is broken into nine subdimensions (daily routine, social functioning, intellectual functioning, emotional functioning, economic status, health status, well-being, life satisfaction, and symptoms related to the disease under study as well as other diseases). Comprehensive rationales have also been provided to justify the inclusion of each of these quality of life criterion.

However, before proceeding to analyse further the plethora of definitions and approaches to quality of life it may useful in the context of health services to discuss more closely the concept of health. Ware (1991) has suggested that we should begin by looking at the two dimensions of life, namely its quantity and its quality. Quantity can be indicated in terms of the length of one's life, life expectancy and mortality rates, but Ellinson (1979) has pointed out that these indices have little value in capturing the quality of years lived in developed countries.

What is required are more qualitative indices. Consequently a comprehensive view of one's health has often been equated with the quality of one's life. But is this a valid assumption? Quality of life surely encompasses much more that the status of one's health. For instance, issues such as standard of living, quality of housing, the district in which one lives and job satisfaction are frequently included in quality of life definitions and scales.

However, contemporary approaches to defining health go beyond objective states such as death and the extent of morbidity. Broader conceptualizations of health include how well a person functions in everyday life, his/her emotional well-being, and self-reports of health in general. Hence "quality of life" has been adopted as a way of summarizing a set of qualitative indices that go far beyond the traditional clinical approach to defining health status. This approach is not without its problems, because it is obviously too inclusive. While jobs, housing, schools and the neighborhood are related to one's functional status and overall well-being, they are not strictly components of one's health.

Nevertheless, the multidimensionality of health is recognized in the definition of health suggested by the World Health Organization (WHO, 1948, 1958). The WHO defined health as a "state of complete physical, psychological and social well-being and not merely the absence of disease or infirmity". This definition goes beyond the traditional medical model which seeks only the cure or the palliation of disease. In an endeavour to restrict the breadth of the quality of life concept and to make it more amenable for use in clinical trials Fries and Spitz (1991) developed a hierarchical model which concentrated upon "health status" and "patient outcome." An assumption is made that these constructs constitute "quality of life." Health status is seen as a measure of quality of life at a particular point in time while patient outcome refers to a final health status measurement taken after the application of treatment(s) and/or the passage of time. In this model health outcomes have been restricted to five dimensions; a patient's desire to be alive as long as possible; to function normally; to be free of pain and other physical, psychological or social symptoms; to be free of iatrogenic problems from the treatment regimen; and to remain economically viable.

In this model five dimension (death, disability, discomfort, drug side-effects, and dollar cost) are seen as mutually exclusive and collectively exhaustive; together defining patient outcome. It is obvious that this approach does not fit comfortably with the broader biopsychosocial approach suggested above. Furthermore, it is apparent that the health outcomes approach is predicated upon the assumption that quality of life indices should be restricted to strictly objective rather than subjective dimensions in order to satisfy scientific rigour.

Another way of approaching the conceptual framework for studying quality of life is to ask the question why should it be studied or used. From a patient's perspective the obvious answer is to improve the effectiveness of his/her treatment. From the therapy level quality of life trials may differentiate between the effects alternative therapies have upon survival or upon different types of disease. Studies may also be conducted to compare two different treatment approaches, for instance using either surgery or a drug to treat a disease. Other uses include commercial interest, especially those of pharmaceutical companies. The prescribing habits of physicians are affected and these in turn impact upon the drugs carried by individual pharmacies. In the area of cancer treatment, in particular, quality of life data, especially the patient's reporting of his/her own perception of level of function, has been used to monitor the palliative and curative effects drugs and their toxic side-effects (Schipper *et al.*, 1984). Quality of life assessments are also being considered as indices to accelerate the approval processes for the use of new drugs (Shoemaker *et al.*, 1990). From the perspective of a country quality of life data are being used to determine the allocation of the health dollar.

A factor which leads to confusion when one addresses the way quality of life has been conceptualized in the health field is the tendency by some to treat specific domains within a multidimensional model as though that domain represented a good index of quality of life. For instance, if one were to adopt Spilker's (1990) suggestion that quality of life generally includes the four categories of (a) physical status and functional abilities, (b) psychological status and well-being, (c) social interactions, and (d) economic status and factors, it is apparent when analysing the literature that many authors who claim to be dealing with quality of life issues are, in reality, only studying one of these domains.

It is obvious that the concept of quality of life in the health field, and indeed in other fields, has been used very loosely without a clear definition and without a coherent theoretical base (Parmenter, 1988, 1992). For instance, Andrews and Withey, as early as 1976, noted that the notion of measuring quality of life could include the measurement of practically anything of interest to anybody. Schipper *et al.* (1990, p. 11) have suggested that "the rubric has become a catcall for inconsistently designed trials, many of which have unclear goals". Schipper *et al.* cited as an example of conceptual confusion a case where an investigator may focus on the rate of wound healing, or sexuality or financial concerns, and then correlate those variables directly with quality of life. While these individual variables may be important factors in a patient's quality of life, without a sound conceptual basis for quality of life, it is very difficult to draw any firm conclusions about his/her overall function when analysing a specific variable.

The paradigmatic shift in the way society is thinking about issues and solving problems related to people with disabilities provided an under-pinning for Schalock's (1991) development of his model of quality of life. Schalock suggested that a model of quality of life should encompass both aspects of the macrosystem that represents cultural trends and factors in society and aspects of the microsystem that relate to the individual (e.g. family, schooling, rehabilitation programs). In the health field a similar paradigm shift may be noted. For instance, Schipper *et al.* (1990, p. 11) have argued that a conceptual formulation has emerged, "which defines quality of life functionally by patients' perception of performance in four areas: physical and occupational function, psychologic state, social interaction and somatic sensation". This is quite a dramatic shift in emphasis for the medical world that formerly operated under what might be termed a "beneficence model" of health care, which assumed that health professionals are best placed to determine what promotes or protects the best interests of the patient. McCullough (1984) has contrasted this model with the "autonomy model" which acknowledges that patients can provide knowledge about what is in their best interests.

This approach is reminiscent of George Engel's tribute to the work of Arthur Schmale, Professor Emeritus of Onclogy in Psychiatry at the University of Rochester School of Medicine and Dentistry. Schmale, suggested Engel (1991, p. 64)

... exemplifies the scientist who seems always to have sensed the appropriateness of looking inward as well as outward. And in no scientific endeavour is the necessity to look inward so obvious, and so ignored, as in clinical medicine. After all, gaining information about a patient's state of health depends not only on having the patient look inward, but also on the doctor's looking inward to evaluate what the patient is reporting.

It is somewhat ironic that medicine from its very beginnings in the clinical study of one person by another depended upon the triad of observation, introspection and dialogue. The advent of 17th century natural science, suggested Engel (1990) relegated introspection and dialogue to a nonscientific status. However, current qualitative approaches to scientific enquiry emphasis the standards of accuracy, completeness, and reproducibility. Increasingly, the exclusive application of the methodologies of the "hard sciences" to answering questions raised in the complex interactions that occur in the study of the human condition is being critically examined.

The inclusion of subjective variables within the formulation of quality of life indices, while more readily accepted in the nonmedical world, have not been received as enthusiastically in the medical arena. Historically physicians have viewed with suspicion the subjective assessment of treatment outcomes by the patient. While the reasons for this are varied, one of the major reasons is the view that the process of medical research should be in keeping with the rigorous application of the Scientific Method.

Early approaches to the concept of quality of life as an outcome parameter in the health sciences were solely empirically driven. Schipper *et al.* (1990) have observed that efforts have been made to develop a conceptual definition of quality of life. They have proposed that five concepts have emerged which add to our current understanding: the psychological approach; the time trade-off or utility concept; Ware's (1984) community-centred concept; the reintegration concept; and Calman's (1984) Gap Principle.

The Psychological View

The psychological view is best epitomized by the call by Engel (1978, 1980) for the inclusion of psychosocial parameters when considering the effects of disease. From a psychological perspective quality of life represents the patient-perceived effects of disease (e.g. "I feel ill"). Here a distinction needs to be made between illness and disease. Illness is what the patient experiences as a result of a particular disease. Physicians concentrate more upon the process of the disease, although there is growing evidence for a direct relationship between the patient's psychosocial response to symptoms and the etiology and treatment of some diseases. Even where this relationship is not evident, physicians are increasingly taking into account the patient's psychosocial response to disease in their treatment regimen.

The Utility Concept

This concept refers to the trade-offs we might make between quantity and quality of life, an approach derived from decision theory. When given the choice between treatments, one which may prolong life, but with an attendant loss of function or impairment; and another which may retain that function, but at the cost of a shorter life, many people with serious diseases will opt for the latter course. The utility concept is somewhat like an accident insurance policy which places a monetary value on a limb or any eye, etc. Good examples are found in McNeil *et al.* (1981) and Torrance (1987).

The utility approach can also be used within an economic framework, especially when there is a need to discriminate between individuals when making clinical judgements about the withholding or withdrawing treatments. For instance quality of life data could tip the balance when the physician is faced with a decision based on the scarcity of resources. At present while there is still debate as to the reliability and/or validity of quantitative quality of life measures it may be somewhat premature to use these data when making decisions between individuals.

The ethical rather than technical concerns the use of such data in clinical decision-making was highlighted in an Ontario study by Till (1986) and Ciampi *et al.* (1982). In this study, 226 females in two Ontario cities were asked their opinions about a hypothetical medical decision concerning whether to use a radical or conservative treatment for a form of malignant lymphoma. The results indicated that the majority of respondents advocated the more radical treatment for those patients who came form a vulnerable group such as those with either disabilities, social isolation or lacking a motivation to improve their situation. The disturbing implication is that this finding is reminiscent of those situations in the past where vulnerable groups in the community (e.g. institutionalized people such as those with mental retardation, mental illness or prisoners) have been exploited by being exposed to risky radical treatments.

Another ethical implication is that marginal groups in society who are not valued highly could have treatments withheld while others whose situations are assessed more favourably could be given the treatment. The social justice implications of this approach will be taken up later.

The utility approach has found more favour among program educators and health policy decision makers. Here the questions revolve not around individuals, but groups requiring especially expensive treatments. Cost-utility analysis is used to relate the cost of an intervention to the number of quality-adjusted life-years (QALYs) gained through the application of intervention. A QALY assumes a year of healthy life expectancy to be worth 1, but regards a year of unhealthy life expectancy as less than 1. As Lee and Miller (1990) have pointed out, QALYs essentially measure the cost effectiveness of specific medical interventions for decision-making at a macro or micro level. Torrance (1986) provided an example (in 1983 dollars) where it was estimated that the cost per QALY gained is $4500 for neonatal intensive care for 1000 to 1499 gram neonates and $54 000 for hospital hemodialysis. Ethical and methodological issues surrounding the use of QALYs will also be raised later.

Ware's Community-Centred Concept

Ware (1984, 1991) has proposed a model which organizes health status and quality of life variables in such a way that a sense of the impact an illness has upon the broader community is given. In this approach Ware has grouped specific variables in concentric circles starting with biological functioning and spreading out in turn to general well-being and behaviour or social/role functioning. He suggested that measures of biological phenomena cannot alone be used to portray human phenomena. In his explication of the model Ware has indicated that it may be possible to use differential weightings for the component parts of the model quality of life construct. Also implicit in the model is the notion that an individual's illness impacts upon the general community. The economic aspects of this proposition have been long recognized, but the impact serious illness or trauma through accident has upon family functioning is often overlooked by health professionals.

The Reintegration Concept

Wood and Williams (1987) building on a model which they referred to as "reintegration to normal living", developed a scale which included the following domains: mobility, self-care, daily activities, recreational activities, family roles, personal relationships, presentation of self, and general coping skills. Underpinning this model was the concept that a person with a chronic disease for which no cure is expected would learn to live with that fact and would get on with their life. There was also a strong element of self-determination implicit in this model. They suggested that for the individual there would be a recognization of his/her physical, psychological, and social characteristics into a harmonious whole, so that after an incapacitating illness or trauma normal living can be resumed.

Two subscales which were developed were found to correlate moderately with Spitzers' Quality of Life Index (Spitzer, *et al.*, 1981), a popular quality of life scale used in the area of oncology. This finding is not surprising for the Spitzer Index samples the domains of activity, daily living, health, support and outlook which coincide fairly closely with those of Wood and Williams.

Calman's Gap Principle

One way of viewing quality of life is to estimate the gap between a patient's expectations and his/her achievements, a position adopted by Calman (1984) whose study of the quality of life of cancer patients revealed that the gap between expectations and achievement varies over time. As the patient's health improves or digresses as a result of treatment or the natural progression of the disease so does their expectations of how they might function. Calman further suggested that "the impact of illness" on patients varied according to how they perceived their quality of life at the time. Thus a person whose illness had caused debilitating effects may have reduced their expectations accordingly.

This approach has value for it introduces the notion of comparing quality of life against some standard, in this case the patient's own expectations. Another way of looking at the gap principle is to compare the patient's actual achievements with his/her potential achievements as estimated by a third party. A number of studies have shown that despite assessments of good potential achievements, patients' estimate of their quality of life have been negative (Andrews and Stewart, 1979; Powell and Powell, 1987). In this respect it is necessary to attempt to increase the patient's awareness of their potential so they may enjoy a higher quality of life. It must be recognized, however, that there is a great variation in the way individuals react to serious illnesses and consequently their perception of their quality of life.

Schipper *et al.* (1990) have rejected a definition of quality of life based upon the World Health Organization's definition of health as being too inclusive 'of elements that are beyond the purview of traditional, apolitical medicine' (p. 16). Instead they have proposed that "Quality of Life" represents the functional effect of an illness and its consequent therapy upon a patient, as perceived by the patient' (p. 16). It is their contention that this definition reflects the goal of medicine which is to reduce and possibly eliminate the morbidity and mortality of a particular disease.

Shumaker *et al.* (1990) have defined quality of life 'as individuals' overall satisfaction with life and their general sense of personal well-being' (p. 96). They have suggested somewhat similar dimensions to those of Schipper *et al.* (1990) and have proposed that six dimensions determine a person's quality of life; the first four including cognitive, social, physical and emotional functioning. Personal productivity or the degree to which a person is able to contribute to society (e.g. through a meaningful paid or unpaid activity) is postulated as a fifth dimension. The final dimension is intimacy, including sexual functioning, but also the giving and receiving of a broad range of behaviours that underlie the presence of a strong relationship with significant others.

This latter dimension is often ignored in other conceptual approaches to quality of life. However, it is one of the central features of the definition proposed by Powers and Goode (cited in Goode, 1990) who have suggested that 'quality of life is primarily a product of relationships between people in each life setting' (p. 43). The importance of the environment or the immediate macrosystem surrounding the individual to his/her quality of life has been strongly emphasized by Goode (1987), and highlights the narrowness of the definitions employed in medicine.

The approach adopted by Fretwell (1990) in her analysis of standards of care for the frail elderly has captured aspects of the "person-environmental fit" approach adopted in the psychological and sociological literature. For instance she has suggested that, 'as human age, there is a continuous interaction of environmental and genetic factors that accentuates the uniqueness of each person' (p. 225). This is consistent with Lipowski's views (1969) who remarked that 'how a person experiences the pathological process, what it means to him (her), and how this meaning influences his (her) behaviour and interaction with others are all integral components of disease viewed as a total human response' (p. 1198).

In discussing the quality of life in the context of persons with a congenital physical or intellectual disability Parmenter (1988, 1992) suggested that the theory of symbolic-interactionism could profitably form a conceptual basis. Fundamental to this approach is the principle that human experiences are mediated by interpretation (Bogdan and Kugelmass, 1984). Another basic element is that the "self" arises and is maintained in a symbolic and interactive world. For people with a congenital disability, and, it is suspected , for those with a serious disease, the development of the self or their identity as a person is influenced from two sources. One comes from outside and proceeds from the social order. The other comes from within and relates to what they can or cannot do. Thus as the same time they have to deal with the negative aspects of their personal condition and cope with the possible negative effects of how they are viewed by significant others. From a philosophical point of view there is a conflict between the existential nature of the person and the social nature of human experience. Using this framework Parmenter (1988) suggested that 'quality of life represents the degree to which individuals have met their needs to create own meanings so they can establish and sustain a viable self in the social world' (p. 15).

This approach is in sympathy with Fava (1990) who saw quality of life as a common pathway for the 'various interlocking mechanism at the neurophysiological, biochemical, experimental and behavioural levels' (p. 71). Fava urged a holistic approach in considering quality of life in relation to disease; one which shifted from a purely biomedical approach that included parameters such as psychological distress, illness, behaviour, and social functioning to one which included the additional psychosocial correlates of illness. Fava made an extremely cogent contribution by stressing the need to consider a person's quality of life *before* the full-blown onset of disease. Such consideration, he suggested, should include issues such as environmental factors associated with the disease, life changes or life events prior to the onset of illness and the occurrence of psychological distress in the preliminary stages of illness.

Siegrist and Junge (1990) in their conceptual approach towards the social dimension of treatment-related subjective health have argued for a stronger recognition of the importance of the social dimension in measures of subjective health, despite Torrance's (1987, p. 594) assertion that 'social functioning is "beyond the skin" and . . . is not an appropriate aspect of health-related quality of life'. Siegrist and Junge have highlighted the social performance and social well-being as being critical aspects of the definition of subjective health. Social performance includes role performance and social skills; the former may be related to formal roles such as resumed vocational activity or informal roles such as membership of clubs or social groups. Social skills are those personal requirements for successful role performance and include sociability, empathy and social interactions. Their description of social well being which includes the four conceptual scales of 'sense of belonging', 'intimacy and trust', social approval' and 'meaningful contribution' has significant parallels with the argument proposed by Parmenter (1988, 1992) above concerning the palpable role that the development of one's identity plays in the conceptual basis of quality of life.

One of the difficulties experienced in most attempts to conceptualize and quality of life is the omission of any consideration of the individual meaning of illness. Few scales of QOL include the opportunity for respondents to rate the significance of particular items to their perception of their quality of life.[1] This highly individualistic phenomena concerning a person's well-being and general life satisfaction almost ensure that most conceptual approaches will be invalid for some people. Mayou (1990) working in the context of cardiovascular disease has stressed this weakness in most approaches to the measurement of quality of life. He cited the example of the uncertain significance of rates of return to work, especially for those of late middle-age. Return to work can be seen by some as a good outcome whilst others may see failure to return to work as an excellent outcome. The use of scales which do not accommodate these individual differences will invalidate much of the findings in quality of life research. This issue will be taken up in more detail in the next section.

An examination of the conceptual bases for much of the study of quality of life in relation to disease has revealed a fairly pragmatic and empirical approach. There is little in the way of solid theory that can be used to generate research hypotheses that might allow one to expand the boundaries of our knowledge base. The most fruitful approaches are those that recognize the interaction between the person with the disease with his/her environment. The recognition of the need to study quality of life from the perspective of the patient is well established as is the need to include psychosomatic aspects. However, there has been an illusion of simplicity that has caused many researches to believe that the measurement of quality of life is simple and feasible. What is required is a more comprehensive and broadened conceptualization of quality of life, one that recognizes the significance of individual meaning. It is essential that models be established that include specific measures of quality of life that are chosen as being of particular importance to patients.

C. SPECIFIC POPULATIONS AND APPROACHES TO MEASUREMENT OF QUALITY OF LIFE

This section will review the use of a number of assessment approaches that have been developed to estimate quality of life in the context of specific populations with serious health problems. The areas covered do not purport to represent the wealth of research and literature available. However, a number of methodological and conceptual problems will be raised that do reflect the current status of quality of life research.

Selection of Quality Of Life Measures In Clinical Trials And Practice

Before selecting an appropriate QOL scale a useful strategy is to ask a number of questions concerning why the assessment is required. Osoba *et al.* (1991) have proposed an algorithm, or set of guidelines, that will help in the selection of the most appropriate measure for assessing quality of life in specific clinical situations. Their algorithm contains four basic questions:

(i) Will the measure be used for screening or case finding?

(ii) Will the measure be used for the obtaining quality of life health profiles?

(iii) Will the measure be used for the assessment of preferences?

(iv) Will the measure be used in clinical decision making?

Hence the purpose for which the data are required will influence to a great degree the nature of the scale adopted.

Among additional questions raised by Osoba *et al.* (1991) concerning scale selection were the following:

(i) Which method of measurement is most appropriate for the purpose?

Here the options are between structured or unstructured interviews and questionnaires that may be either self-assessment or observer-assessment.

(ii) What is the scope of the assessment?

This refers to whether the issues to be covered are general or specific regardless of the method adopted. General assessment contains several dimensions of quality of life while the specific approach focuses upon a single dimension or social aspect within one dimension.

(iii) Are reliable, valid measures available?

Having chosen the purpose of the exercise one needs to explore the psychometric properties of available scales. If none is appropriate a decision has to be made as to whether it is cost effective to design and validate a new instrument.

The major properties of a psychometrically sound instrument are its reliability and validity. In terms of reliability the scale should be internally consistent, have sound test-retest stability and have high inter-rater reliability.

Validity is tested in variety of ways. An instrument should be responsible to changes in quality of life over time. It should also be able to detect differences between groups of patients in differing situations. It is important that a scale have face validity; that is the item should logically apply to the group being assessed. For instance, a number of scales have been developed for specific populations such as those with chronic illnesses (e.g. cancer) and those with psychiatric disorders. It would be unwise to use a scale for a population where the items are logically inappropriate.

There are rigorous statistical techniques available that can be applied to assess the reliability and validity of instruments. These have traditionally been used to demonstrate the scientific rigour of this area of research. For instance Osaba *et al.* (1991) have provided a comprehensive psychometric analysis of a selection of QOL measures developed for cancer patients. The trends towards a more qualitative approach to QOL assessments does not preclude the need, as suggested by Engel (1990, p. 67) for data 'to satisfy standards of accuracy, completeness and reproducibility; claims of proof must conform to rules of evidence and procedures (must) meet the requirements for consensual validation and public accountability.'

(iv) Are the results or outcomes of the assessment meaningful?

Here one has to distinguish between statistical and practical significance. A result may be statistically significant, but have little meaning in a clinical sense. A typical example of this is when large sample sizes are based in randomized clinical trials. Very small group differences in quality of life outcomes will often reach the standard levels of statistical significance, but these results may have little clinical relevance.

Osaba *et al.* (1991) have suggested that researchers should specify the nature of quality-of-life outcomes that will be considered clinically meaningful at the beginning of a study rather than in a *post hoc* manner. They have also highlighted the very important need for researchers not to dismiss findings that have been acknowledged with sound instruments and that are counter-intuitive on a clinical basis. They cited cases in cancer studies where results have run contrary to *a priori* expectations, requiring a serious reappraisal of conventional thinking. Medicine is not the only area where scientists need to reexamine existing paradigms.

The following examination of a approaches to quality of life assessment in the areas of cardiovascular disorders, oncology, and rehabilitation, is illustrative of the conceptual and measurement difficulties that surround this topic.

Cardiovascular Disorders

In this area research has explored five main issues: (a) description and understanding of the effects of different types of cardiac disorder upon all aspects of quality of life; (b) the relationship between effects on quality of life and physical impairment; (c) individual variation in response to cardiac disorder; (d) the design of interventions to prevent and treat medically unnecessary psychosocial problems, and (e) the evaluation of interventions; medical, surgical, educational and psychological.

As in other illnesses, two approaches may be utilized in the measurement of quality of life. One can use *general (or generic) measures* which are standardized and are applied widely to these without different types of illness for purposes of comparison. These measures usually provide either a health profile with subscales for different aspects of social functioning which can be aggregated. Alternatively the scales produce a single figure index which is often used in cost benefit analyses.

Mayou (1990) has argued that these general measures have a role 'as long as they are not seen as a simple unconsidered answer to the need to be seen to be measuring quality of life' (p. 103). General measures will often not reveal important clinical changes because they are usually too 'broad brush' to detect specific problems of particular illnesses. A related problem is irrespective of whether one uses general or specific measures, quality of life research has overly concentrated upon overall changes within groups of patients and has obscured the significance of individual variation. This highlights the need to use quality of life instruments as process measures as well as an index of final outcomes. What are required are well-chosen *specific measures*. In this case it is best to start asking basic questions of the patients and their families as to what they feel is important in their life quality. For instance, what are their particular problems? What are their expectations concerning treatment? These aspects of quality of life seldom appear in the popular general measures of health status.

As a result of the popularity of general measures, Stewart *et al.* (1989) pointed out that there has been an underestimation of the clinical and economic significance of including psychological aspects of quality of life in both acute and chronic heart disease. Studies have concentrated on "common sense" measures of functional status and on employment outcomes while ignoring in large measure the mental state of patients. This raises the issue of the reluctance of researchers to accept the validity of "soft" psychological measures.

Nevertheless, there has been a perceptible trend towards a greater inclusion of patient involvement in studies concerned with cardiovascular disorders. For example, in a comprehensive review in 1984 of those areas of psychological and social functioning which should be assessed in trials of cardiovascular treatment elements, Wenger *et al.* (1984) did not include aspects which related to a patient's feelings of satisfaction, frustration, anger, excessive caution, expectations, etc. By 1990, however, Wenger and Furberg (1990) had moved their position to that of strong support for the inclusion of patient life satisfaction factors such as well-being, emotional state, perceptions and expectations. They argued strongly, too, that the impact of the disease upon the family and significant others should be taken into account. They noted that 'the perceptions of the patients and their families reflect their personal value system and judgments regarding general health status, well-being, and life satisfaction' (p. 337)

The importance of assessing patient and family expectations is of particular importance where those expectations are excessively limited. The effectiveness of new therapies which can improve the outlook for both morbidity and mortality may be curtailed because of limited expectations brought about by the course of the illness.

A popular outcome index for cardiovascular treatments has been return to work, so much so that it has almost become a 'surrogate for quality of life' (Wenger and Furberg, 1990, p. 338). As noted above, Mayou (1990) found return to work as an unreliable quality of life index for arterial surgery. In those severely impaired or elderly, return to paid work is an unreasonable goal of most interventions and should not be seen as an aspect of quality of life. A patient's perceptions of health status and his/her ability to work, rather than objective measures of functional capability, are more often the determinant of whether the person returns to paid employment.

Returning to the question whether to use general or specific measures of quality of life it can be argued that even disease-specific indices are not sensitive to the variations in the stages or severity of the illness. For example, attributes of quality of life for coronary patients may be different across the various stages of the treatment and subsequent recovery. There would also be different areas of concern for a patient with a stable angina pectoris compared with one who has acute myocardial infarction.

There is a large body of literature on the psychological consequences of treatment following myocardial infarction. The seminal work by Hackett and Cassem (1984) at The Massachusetts General Hospital in the 1960s gave rise to much of this work. There is evidence that the major consequences for social functioning in areas such as leisure activities, social and family life and sexual activities are not closely related to ongoing physical problems (Mayou, 1979). Further, these various areas of mental and social functioning are not necessarily highly related either. This calls for a broader approach to evaluation.

In the heart transplant area there have been reports of the considerable benefits to quality of life for patients in addition, of course, to their life expectancy (Buxton et al., 1985) as assessed by the Nottingham Health Profile. Mayou (1990) has suggested, however, that the complexity of the consequences of a heart transplant are not revealed by a very simple measure of quality of life. For instance, Mai et al. (1986) and Shapiro and Kornfeld (1989) have highlighted the presence of significant psychiatric, social and family problems in this population. Such studies do not question the success of heart transplants, but they do alert us to the psychological and social support needs of patients and their families. This is further support for the need of a more comprehensive assessment of quality of life and health status.

Raczynski and Oberman (1990) have summed up the position admirably with their suggestion that one of the key factors that mediates the disability effects on quality of life of people with cardiovascular problems is the patient's learning the disability role. In the majority of QOL assessment scales little attention is paid to the effects disability may have upon the individual's definition of him/her self as a person and his/her role in the social environment. There is a clear need to shift the focus in this area from longitudinal research that uses overly simplistic outcome indices, to research that seeks to maximize and maintain the many facets of quality of life. This will require a wider range of instruments which include interview-based as well as self-report approaches. Mayou (1990, p. 107) has put the case rather pungently in his suggestion that 'such changes in methodology will be impossible without acceptance that quality of life is not a simple, cheap and dubious extra, but a subject deserving as much attention as physical outcome measures'.

Quality Of Life In Oncology Patients[2]

Of all diseases cancer possibly invokes the most profound fear in persons so inflicted (in more recent years, however, AIDS may have eclipsed the fear that a diagnosis of cancer evokes). Not only do the majority of the 100 or more separate disease identified as cancer result in a significant threat to life, but many are accompanied by severe pain and suffering. Further, there are often disastrous side effects associated with any of the treatments which have led to a focus on 'quality of survival'.

The main themes that have merged in quality of life research in oncology have been: (a) the evaluation of therapies, including psychosocial criteria; (b) the provision of a better basis for decisions between competing treatments by including criteria of quantity and quality of survival, and (c) the development of more focussed and more efficient ways of psychosocial support for patients with malignant diseases.

The types of quality of life assessments used in cancer studies have included: (a) population-based assessments, such as the Quality of Well-

Being Index (Bush, 1984) and the Sickness Impact Profile (Bergner *et al.*, 1981); (b) psychosocial assessments of coping (Derogatis, 1986) and depression (Beck *et al.* (1961); (c) global measures such as quality of life adjusted years (QALY) (Weinstein, 1983) and time without symptoms or toxicity (TWIST) (Gelber and Goldhirsch, 1986); (d) functional indices including the Karnofsky Index (Karnofsky *et al.*, 1948) and the World Health Organization Scales (WHO) (Zubrod *et al.*, 1960); and (e) multidimensional instruments such as the Functioning Living Index for Cancer (FLIC) (Schipper *et al.*, 1984), Quality of Life Index (Spitzer *et al.*, 1981) and the Padilla Quality of Life Index (QLI) (Padilla *et al.*, 1983).

The low correlations found between objective and subjective indices of quality of life outlined by Lewis and Ryan (1986) in their community studies are supported by the findings of Muthny *et al.* (1990) that there is not a high relationship between medical parameters and quality of life scores. The low psychophysiological correlations found in persons who are chronically ill may be explained by their coping behaviours that include cognitive, emotional and behavioural efforts to overcome the stress and achieve adaptation to the sequence of the illness. It has been observed that cancer patients report better qualities of life than would be expected for an independent assessment of the impact of their disease and its treatments. De Haes and von Knippenbert (1985) have suggested that a patient's response may be a reflection of perceptual restructuring where the patient who expecting less, feels that he or she is doing well. The adaptation theory of Helson and Bevan (1967) would account for this phenomenon. Alternatively, a more psychopathological stance taken by Hurny *et al.* (1987) suggests that patients tend to respond in a socially desirable way, especially as they age.

An early, yet significant, contribution to the quality of life literature by Campbell *et al.* (1976) was their observation that a quality of life judgement contains both cognitive and affective components, each of which can change independently of the other. For example, when patients indicate that they remain satisfied they may be masking the negative affective changes which are occurring concurrently. This will require further independent assessment. The role that cognition plays and the independent effects of the effective components of quality of life require further intensive study, particularly in the context of providing adequate psychosocial support for patients with cancer, or indeed other illnesses that are surrounded by severe emotional stresses.

For instance, in the area of chronic obstructive pulmonary disease, Jensen (1983) found that social support and life stress predicted the number of hospitalizations better than did the patients's demographic characteristics, the severity of the illness, or previous hospitalization. Several studies have revealed the significance of instrumental and emotional support provided by spouses, friends and relatives to a person's quality of life and their response to treatment. Economic security has also been found to predict better adaptation (Sexton and Munro, 1988; Young, 1982).

A fruitful avenue for further studies is an examination of the effects an individual's coping strategies may have upon quality of life outcomes with respect to physical functioning, family/partnership relationships, emotional well-being, and social and occupational functioning. The role that social support may play in this process also requires investigation. These questions would obviously involve an interdisciplinary approach involving oncologists, psychologists and psychotherapists. It is anticipated that the quality of life cancer patients can be improved not only by medical interventions, but also by more effective doctor-patient relationships wherein diagnosis and possible treatments are better communicated to the patient. A further important consideration is the improvement of psychosocial care including the effective support of an individual's coping processes. This calls for an individual-specific approach to the assessment of quality of life.

Rehabilitation

Despite the shift of emphasis from a narrowly focussed compensatory program to one which seeks to reintegrate persons with disabilities into community life, assessment of rehabilitation outcomes rely heavily upon objective functional indices which ignore to a large extent the subjective aspects of a person's life. While the term rehabilitation is used generically in the disability literature, encompassing programs for people with congenital impairment, usually referred to as developmental disabilities, and for those whose disabilities have been acquired through accident or disease, this review will be restricted to programs for the latter group.

In any examination of rehabilitation outcomes one is struck by the absence of references to theory. As in other areas of health services this omission reflects the lack of well-elaborated theories of rehabilitation and disablement. Having its genesis in medicine, rehabilitation has been overly influenced by the need to define outcomes specifically and objectively within the rubric of the "hard" sciences. A related influence has been the need to restrict outcomes or goals to those aspects that the rehabilitation professional can directly control. The nature of much of the rehabilitation industry, relying heavily on third-party sponsors, also does not encourage the evaluation of the long-term effects of rehabilitation services. These factors, together with the difficulties of assessing the influence of environmental variables, often beyond the control of rehabilitation professionals, may explain the absence of a sound conceptual base for the rehabilitation process. This in turn has retarded the development of research programs which address the broader, and often more subjective, elements of quality of life.

The pervasive influence of the independent living paradigm (De Jong, 1981), the growth of disabilities studies in which people with disabilities are speaking out (Finkelstein, 1980; Stoddard, 1978; Vash, 1984); and the influence of the literature on the social construction of disability (Barton, 1989; Fulcher, 1989; Söder, 1984), have all contributed to a broader perspective on the outcomes of rehabilitation programs.

The paradigm that has led to the development of a more integrated model of rehabilitation than the earlier emphasis upon observable pathology and dysfunction is the World Health Organization classification of impairment and handicap (Wood, 1975). Grange and Gresham (1984) have presented a model wherein concepts are organized across three levels: organ, person and society. Within each of these the condition results directly or indirectly, in either impairment, disability or handicap. This framework allows for functional assessments of physical performance, mental performance, emotional performance, and social performance (Jette, 1984).

While there have been conceptual advances in the delivery and assessment of rehabilitation programs, the field has been slow to incorporate the impact of disability upon the psychosocial functioning of the person. One gains the impression from a review of the literature that the rehabilitation field is still dominated by the various professional groups which deliver the services, despite Turner's (1990, p. 249) suggestion that measurement of rehabilitation outcomes is moving from 'situation and institution-specific scale development to broader-based, coordinated, interdisciplinary work.' Ellwood (1988), for instance, called for the development of an outcome management system which would have quality of life assessment as its core.

However, rehabilitation counselling has made a significant contribution to the study of quality of life. For instance, Roessler (1990) has presented a quality of life perspective on rehabilitation counselling which integrates competing program goals such as client independence or employment into higher order, multidimensional rehabilitation outcomes. He noted that counsellors committed to the quality of life orientation work from a wellness and holistic position that addresses both the development of the individual and the environment in which the person lives.

An interesting study by Scherer (1988) illustrated an important aspect of quality of life for people with spinal cord injuries or cerebral palsy. She compared the use or nonuse of assistive devices by these two groups. The users of both disabilities saw their quality of life as being within their control, whereas nonusers believed otherwise. Despite numerous methodological problems in assessing locus of control, persons assessed as having an internal locus of control appear to have more than a coincidental power over their disabilities. It seems that it is this power that can make the difference in a person's prognosis and quality of life (Evans, 1991). It would appear that an important dimension in rehabilitation outcome studies is the degree to which the persons feel in control of their lives.

A related issue is professionalism which defines the hierarchical relationship between the health care worker and the patient. The traditional dominance of the former over the latter is giving way to a more equal partnership, or indeed in some situations, a complete reversal of power. An interesting study by Lomas *et al.* (1987) illustrated the differences in values between clinicians and a group of patients with language disabilities. Clinicians and patients generated lists of important functional communication situations to develop a measure of quality of life. Results indicated that the clinicians underestimated the patient's focus on social needs. The clinician-generated items were not fully representative of patient values.

The trend in quality of life studies in the area of traumatic brain injury (TBI) has been toward the assessment of psychosocial variables such as those related to family relationships (Brooks, 1992) and empowerment (Jacobs *et al.*, 1990). It is essential, too, for longitudinal studies which can assess changes in quality of life over time. Such assessments can be used for adaptations to lifelong living programming. Indeed the use of quality of life assessments as process as well as outcome measures is to be encouraged. The ultimate success of such programming is measured by lack of institutionalization and by improvement of individual control and quality of life. Increases noted in passive behaviours by people with TBI over time are a cause of concern and require specific attention (Diller and Ben-Yishay, 1987).

In conditions such as TBI and other impairments where recovery to pretrauma states is unlikely, the provision of environmental supports has increasing relevance, especially where the efficacy of treatments is questionable. The inclusion of the concept of support in the recently promulgated definition of mental retardation by the American Association on Mental Retartdation (1992) is a model worthy of consideration for other impairments where handicaps can be reduced through appropriate community support. The roles that friendship networks and close personal relationships play in enhancing quality of life also need to be considered more urgently by rehabilitation services (Knox and Parmenter, 1993).

The life-experience difficulties experienced by people with TBI are not dissimilar to those experienced by people with mental illness. Both groups, because of their emotional and behavioural disorders feel discriminated against and frustrated because of the lack of respect they receive from the community. In a study of 204 persons with serious mental illness, drawn from eleven rehabilitation and mental health centres, Coursey *et al.* (1991) found that the majority of consumers wanted more help with quality of life issues than symptom reduction. They were concerned by their powerlessness and feelings of rejection. Rehabilitation programs that provide an enhancement of economic resources and an empowerment approach to service delivery have also been found to be significantly related to overall quality of life. Perceptions of mastery accounted for the impact of these components of life satisfaction (Rosenfield, 1992).

The diversity of the players in the rehabilitation system and their associated values will continue to influence the types of variables that will be included in outcome studies. Increased emphasis upon the quality of life of people, both in the short and long-term after traumatic injury or illness, may result in the development of a more coherent theory of rehabilitation; one that may lead to new treatment methods which are based upon a more holistic appreciation of human functioning.

D. USES AND ABUSES

Research into the quality of the lives of people who have serious illness or who have experienced traumatic injuries offers a rich area of investigation that can lead to dramatic improvements in the way we deliver health and rehabilitation services. The paradigmatic shifts in the field of disability generally are having profound effects upon service delivery and the way we view the nature of illness and disability and its subsequent amelioration by the various professional groups. In order that"quality of life" as a concept does not become maligned because of its vagueness and/or because it poses supposedly insuperable problems in its accurate measurement, a number of questions will be explored in this concluding section. These questions include the rationale for measuring quality of life; discussions concerning who should measure it; how should it be measured; and what are some of the ethical issues surrounding its measurement?

Rationale

Quality of life indices have been used to assess outcomes of clinical trials, to compare the efficacy of different treatments, to evaluate the cost-utility and cost-effectiveness of health care programs, to assist quality assurance and to assist in the marketing and regulation of drugs.

Assessments of outcomes of clinical trials in cancer patients provide an excellent rationale for including quality of life assessments in addition to biological data such as overall survival, disease-free survival, end-response rates, in addition to haematological and other indices of toxicity. With current interventions there is no guarantee that curing the patient's cancer will return him/her to the same level of quality of life as in the precancer state. Relief of physiological symptoms is not necessarily accompanied by an improvement in quality of life. Taking quality of life considerations into account may allow the patients to make decisions as to whether they wish to undergo specific forms of treatment. Pretreatment states of quality of life may also have prognostic value especially as a stratification variable when designing clinical tests. If quality of life measures used are sensitive to clinically important changes, then the resulting information can alert clinicians to the onset of morbidity associated with a disease. This may allow appropriate preventative measures to be taken.

Health economists have used cost-effective analysis as a means of quantifying the relative benefits of medical procedures. With a cost-effectiveness analysis approach, medical outputs are equated with the number of lives or life-years saved. Thus, a redistribution of funds to projects with a low cost per life can be seen as a means of increasing the total number of life-years that may be gained (Drummond, 1991). A major weakness in the approach was that it treated all life-years as having equal value irrespective of the quality of life (Richardson, 1991). This has raised obvious ethical issues, especially in the treatment of neonates with severe abnormalities (Zaner, 1986).

Perceived weakness in the cost-effectiveness analysis approach has led to the development of the concept of quality-of-life adjusted years (QALYs) (Williams, 1979, 1985).

Administration Of Scales

There are conflicting opinions concerning who should complete QOL scales. Many of the more popular scales are of a self-report nature for ease of administration. Another approach is to use proxy raters. Fava (1990), for instance, have maintained that observer-rated methods, especially when the interviewers are properly trained, provide a far more reliable assessment than self-rated instrments. Another view is that it is the patients who are in the best position to set the standard by which they will assess their present status (Osaba, 1991). Studies have indicated that observers' ratings are consistently lower than patients' ratings. The patients's perception of what is an acceptable standard also changes with time. A case in point is where one patient expects a cure as against one who knows the illness is incurable. The former patient probably has a much higher standard than the latter whose primary concern may be comfort. The optimum path would be to conduct structured interviews where the patients can elaborate upon their responses . Reputable forms of qualitative data analysis techniques can be used to provide both reliable and valid information.

How Should QOL Be Measured?

One of the problems observed in quality of life research is the elusive search for a 'gold standard' scale; one that can be used across populations and one that can be used for a variety of purposes. A good example is the Quality of Life (QL) Index developed by Spitzer *et al.*, in 1981. The authors set out to develop a simple, quantified instrument that would reflect the different dimension of quality of life, somewhat similar to the Apgar scale used with neonates. The scale has proven to be a reliable and valid assessment of an individual's health related quality of life and is responsive to changes in life's quality over time. It has been used extensively with patients with cancer in addition to those with other debilitating disease. It has been administered as a self-report or by proxy raters such as significant others, the physician, or other health care providers. Its prominence and reputation is such that it is frequently used as a validating tool by other investigators developing instruments with similar theoretical bases.

In their initial development of the Index Spitzer and colleagues set up three advisory panels, each of 43 people representing the patients' relatives, health professionals, clergy, and the general public. From structured and unstructured questionnaires, factors that comprised quality of life were determined, together with information on the relative importance of each factor. Draft forms of a scale were developed and tested on a sample of 339 subjects. A final index emerged with five dimensions; activity, daily living, health, support, and outlook. In addition a linear analog scale which assessed the global attributes in quality of life was incorporated plus a ten-item questionnaire (Multiscale) which also assessed quality of life.

Its simplicity of administration and its global nature has resulted in its widespread use across a wide range of objectives. These have included comparisons between continuous and intermittent chemotherapy in cancer patients (Coates *et al.*, 1987); comparisons between patients with end-stage renal failure receiving continuous ambulatory peritoneal, home or self, or hospital dialysis (Churchill *et al.*, 1987); comparisons of day hospital and in-patient management for cancer patients (Mor *et al.*, 1988).; the value of intensive care for critically ill patients (Sage *et al.*, 1986); and the validation of utility assessment (Churchill *et al.*, 1987). A problem with the QL Index is that the domain "social support" may be a correlate, rather than an outcome measure of quality of life. A difficulty experienced here is the lack of clarity of how "social support" is defined. It may include social contacts, which is closer to performance of social rules; as well as social resources which are more analogous to the concept of social support. The former has quite subjective dimensions, while the latter can be assessed more objectively.

A number of conceptual and methodological problems arise when one approaches specific questions using a global measure. For instance, there is evidence in the case of the QL Index that it correlates better with instruments containing elements of physical performances as opposed to psychosocial functioning. Rather than attempting to use a single index as a measure of quality of life it would seem more reasonable to first ask the question 'for what purpose will the data be used' and to design an instrument that does not purport to come up with a single score. As discussed above, many of the global scales fail to take into account the differential weightings individuals place upon certain aspects of their lives.

Whether one gathers "hard" (i.e. objective) data or "soft" (i.e. subjective) data, measurement tools should have the characteristics of reliability, precision, responsiveness and validity. Gathering independent data to establish concurrent validity and demonstrating the reproducibility of results help to establish the validity of quality of life measures. One of the most serious omissions in much of the scale developments has been the paucity of studies that have tested their construct validity against a sound theoretical base.

Ethical Considerations[3]

Two important principles must be borne in mind when assessing the quality of life of patients. The first is that the long-term goal should be to improve the care of patients. This is consonant with the beneficence principle of a physician's obligation to improve the patient's welfare and well-being. The second principle is that one must always respect the autonomy of the patient. Hence the patient's views and priorities must always be paramount. This will require the active participation of the patient in the quality of life assessment process (Beauchamp and Childress, 1989). Bioethical principles should also have a pervasive influence upon the design; review, conduct, interpretation and reporting of the research instruments for assessing quality of life (Till, 1991).

In the area of 'utility-based' quality of life assessments which have their origins in the decision making theory of von Neumann and Morgenstern (1947) a number of possibly unwarranted assumptions are made. This approach which forms the basis of the concept of QALYs relies upon the aggregation of the duration of survival with the quality of survival into a single variable. Two caveats may be made. The first is that the selection of the algorithm to determine the precise aggregation of scores is an arbitrary one. For instance, different weights can be given to the elderly, or the young or people suffering a particular disease. The crucial question is who decides? The second is that people who decide the trade-offs between quality versus quantity decisions are usually not the people suffering the disease.

It is natural that health economists, faced with ever increasing "blow-outs" in health care budgets, seek measures which can ration these services in an equitable manner. However, as currently used, measures of QALYs underestimate the significance of disability and handicaps as compared with life expectancy. Harris (1987) argued that QALYs fallaciously value time lived, instead of individual lives; taking an excessively narrow view of what quality of life might be.

E. CONCLUSION

The literature on quality of life in the medical area reveals a tension between those who would wish to focus on the biomedical aspects of disease and those who take the broader approach; an approach that seeks to open a dialogue between physician and patient. The power of dialogue and introspection has the potential to elucidate more effectively the meaning of quality of life and to enhance the accuracy and validity of information reported. Criticism of the conceptual bases of quality of life research, including overemphasis upon general concepts; the neglect of mental state; the failure to recognize the range of individual responses; the neglect of individual meaning of quality of life; and the neglect of consequence for the family may be ameliorated by a more equal partnership between instrument developers and those being assessed.

Goode (1991) has suggested that addressing what quality of life actually means from an epistemological perspective may be of more value than developing more indices that may manifest theoretical, definitional, operational, and methodological problems. Interestingly, the quest for effective quality of life measures may forge a closer link between those who emphasize the application of biomedical concepts and techniques and those who wish to include psychosocial aspects normally studied by the behavioural and social sciences. This rapprochement and consequent shifts in attitudes may have a greater impact upon health services than quality of life assessments *per se*.

NOTES

[1] A recent Australian scale developed by R. Cummins (1991) provides respondents with the opportunity to weight the significance various items have in respect to their perceptions of QOL.

[2] The reader is referred to Osaba (1991) for a comprehensive analysis of the effect of cancer on quality of life.

[3] For a comprehensive discussion of ethical issues in the disability field the reader should consult Duncan and Woods (eds.) (1989).

REFERENCES

American Association on Mental Retardation: 1992, Mental Retardation. Definition, Classification and Systems of Supports (Author, Washington, D.C.).

Andrews, K. and J. Stewart: 1979, 'He can but does he?', Rheumatology Rehabilitation 18, pp. 43–48.

Andrews, F. M. and S. B. Withey: 1976, Social Indicators of Well-being (Plenum Press, New York).

Barton, L. (ed.): 1989, Disability and Dependency (The Falmer Press, London).

Beauchamp, T. L. and J. F. Childress: 1989, Pinciples of Biomedical Ethics, 3rd ed. (Oxford University Press, New York).

Beck, A. T., C. N. Ward and M. Mendelson et al.: 1961, 'An inventory for measuring depression', Archives General Psychiatry 4, pp. 5611–5671.

Bergner, M., R. A. Babbit, W. B. Carter and B. S. Gibson: 1981, 'The Sickness Impact Profile: Development and final revision of a health care status measure', Medical Care 19, pp. 787–805.

Bogdan, R. and J. Kugelmass: 1984, 'Case studies of mainstreaming. A symbolic interactionist approach to special schooling', cited in L. Barton and S. Tomlinson (eds.), Special Education and Social Interests (Croom Helm, London), pp. 173–191.

Brooks, N.:1992, 'Psychosocial assessment after traumatic brain injury', Scandinavian Journal of Rehabilitation Medium Supplement 26, pp. 126–131.

Bush, J. W.: 1984, 'General health policy model/quality of well-being. (QWB) Scale', in N. K. Wegner, M. E. Matson, C. E. Furberg et al. (eds.), Quality of Life in Clinical Trials of Cardiovascular Therapies (Le Jacq, New York), pp. 189–199.

Buxton, M., R. Acheson, N. Caini, S. Gibson and B. O'Brien: 1985, 'Costs and benefits of the heart transplant programmes at Harefield and Papworth Hospitals' Research Report No. 12 (Department of Health and Social Security, London).

Calman, K. C.: 1984, 'Quality of life in cancer patients – An hypothesis', Journal of Medical Ethics 10, pp. 124–127.

Campbell, A., P. E. Converse and W. L. Rodgers: 1976, The Quality of American Life (Sage, New York).

Churchill, D. N., G. W. Torrance., D. W. Taylor., C. C. Barnes., D. Ludwn., A. Shimizu and E. K. M. Smith: 1987, Clinical Investigative Medicine 10, p. 14.

Ciampi, A., M. Shilberfeld and J. E. Till: 1982, 'Measurement of individual preferences: The importance of "situation specific" variables', Medical Decision Making 2, p. 483.

Coates, A., V. Gebski, J. F. Bishop, P. Jeal, R. C. Woods, R. Snyder, M. H. N. Tollersall, M. Byrne, V. Harvey, G. Gill, J. Simpson, R. Drummond, J. Brown, R. van Cooten and J. F. Forbes: 1987, 'Improving the quality of life during chemotherapy for advanced breast cancer', New England Journal of Medicine 317, p. 1490.

Coursey, R. D., E. W. Farrel and J. H. Zahniser: 1991, 'Consumers' attitudes toward psychotherapy, hospitalization, and aftercare', Health and Social Work 16, pp. 155–161.

Cummins, R: 1991, Comprehensive Quality of Life Scale – Intellectual Disability (ComQol-ID) (Deakin University, Malvern, Australia).

De Haes, J. C. M. and F. C. E. van Knippenberg: 1985. 'The quality of life of cancer patients: A review of the literature', Social Sciences Medicine 20, pp. 809–817.

De Jong, G.: 1981, Environmental Accessibility And Independent Living Outcomes. Directions For Disability Policy And Research (University Centre for International Rehabilitation, Michigan State University).

Derogatis, L. R.: 1986, 'The Psychological adjustment to illness scale (PAIS)', Journal of Psychosomatic Research 30, pp. 77–91.

Diller, L. and Y. Ben-Yisha: 1987, 'Analyzing rehabilitation outcomes of persons with head injury', in M. J. Fuhrer (ed.), Rehabilitation Outcomes: Analysis And Measurement (Paul H. Brookes, Baltimore).

Drummond, M.: 1981, Studies In Economic Appraisal In Health Care (Oxford University Uniting Press, Oxford).

Duncan, B. and D. Woods (eds.): 1989, Ethical Issues In Disability And Rehabilitation. Report of an International Conference of the Society for Disability Studies (World Rehabilitation Fund, Inc, New York).

Einstein, A.: 1950, Out of My Later Years (Philosophical Library, New York).

Ellinson, J.: 1979, 'Introduction to the theme: Socio medical health indicators', in J. Ellinson and A. E. Siegmann (eds.), Socio-Medical Health Indicators (Baywood, Farmindgale, 3, New York).

Ellwood, P. M.: 1985, 'Outcome management: A technology of patient experience', New England Journal of Medicine 318, pp. 1551–1556.

Engel, G. E.: 1978, 'The biopsychosocial model and the education of health professionals', Annals of the New York Academy of Science 310, pp. 169–181.

Engel, G. E.: 1980, 'The clinical application of the biopsychosocial model', American Journal of Psychiatry 13, pp. 535–543.

Engel, G. L.: 1990, 'On looking inward and being scientific. A tribute to Arthur H. Schmale, MD', Psychotherapy and Psychosomatics 54, pp. 63–69.

Evans, J. H.: 1991, The relationship between internal locus of control and rehabilitation prognosis. ED350556.

Fava, G.: 1990, 'Methodological and conceptual issues in research on quality of life', Psychotherapy and Psychometrics 54, pp. 70–76.

Finkelstein, V.: 1980, Attitudes And Disabled People: Issues For Discussion (World Rehabilitation Fund, Inc., New York).

Fretwell, M. D.: 1990, 'The frail elderly: Creating standards of care', in B. Spilker (ed.) Quality of Life Assessments in Clinical Trials (Raven Press, New York), pp. 225–235.

Fries, J. F. and W. P. Spitz: 1991, 'The Hierarchy of patient outcomes', in B. Spilker (ed.), Quality of Life Assessments In Clinical Trials (Raven Press, New York), pp. 25–35.

Fuhrer, M. J.: 1987, 'Overview of outcome analysis in rehabilitation', in M. J. Fuhrer (ed.), Rehabilitation Outcomes. Analysis And Measurement (Brookes Paul H., Baltimore), pp. 1–15.

Fulcher, G.: 1989, Disabling Policies? A Comparative Approach To education Policy And Disability (The Falmer Press, London).

Gilber, R. D. and A. Goldhirsch: 1986, 'A new endpoint for the assessment of adjuvant therapy in post menopausal women with operable breast cancer', Journal of Clinical Oncology 4, pp. 1772–1779.

Goode, D. A.: 1987, The Interim Report Of The Work Group On QOL For Persons With Disabilities (The Mental Retardation Institute, Valhala, N.Y.).

Goode, D. A.: 1990, 'Thinking about and discussing quality of life', in R. L. Schalock (ed.), Quality of Life. Perspectives And Issues (America, Washington, D.C.).

Goode, D. A.: 1991, 'Quality of life research: A change agent for persons with disabilities'. Paper presented to 1991 American Association on Mental Retardation, Washington, D.C.

Granger, C. V. and G. E. Gresham (eds.): 1984, Functional Assessment In Rehabilitation Medicine (Williams and Wilkins, Baltimore).

Hackett, T. D. and N. H. Cassem: 1984, 'Psychological aspects of rehabilitation after myocardial infarction and coronary artery bypass surgery', in N. K. Wenger and H. K. Hellerstein (eds.), Rehabilitation of the Coronary Patient, 2nd edition (Wiley, New York).

Harris, J.: 1987, 'QALLYfying the value of life', Journal of Medical Ethics 13, pp. 117–123.

Helson, H. and W. Bevan :1967, Contemporary Approaches To Psychology (Van Norstrand, Princeton, N.J.).

Hurney, C., F. Poasetski, R. Bagin and J. Holland: 1987, 'High social desirability in patients being treated of advanced colorectal or bladder cancer: Eventual impact on the assessment of quality of life', Journal of Psychosocial Oncology 5, pp. 19–29.

Jacobs, H. E., M. Beatnik and J. V. Sandhorst: 1990, 'What is lifelong living, and how does it relate to quality of life?', Journal of Head Trauma Rehabilitation 5, pp. 1–8.

Jesens, P. S.: 1983, 'Risk protective factors, and supportive interventions in chronic airway obstruction', Archives of General Psychiatry 40, pp. 1203–1207.

Jette, A. M.: 1984, 'Concepts of Health and methodological issues in functional assessment', in C. V. Granger and G. E. Gresham (eds.), Functional Assessment In Rehabilitation Medicine (Williams and Wilkins, Baltimore).

Karnofsky, D. A., W. N. Abelmann, L. F. Crover and J. H. Buchenal: 1948, 'The use of nitrogen mustards in the palliative treatment of carcinoma', Cancer 1, pp. 634–656.

Knox, M. and T. R. Parmenter: 1993, 'Social networks and support networks for people with mild intellectual disability in competitive employment', International Journal of Rehabilitation Research 16, pp. 18–12.

Levine, S. and S. H. Croog: 1984, 'What constitutes quality of life: A conceptualization of the dimensions of life quality in the healthy populations and patients with cardiovascular disease', in N. K. Wegner, M. E. Mattson, C. D. Furberg and J. Elinson (eds.), Assessment of Quality Of Life In Clinical Trials Of Cardiovascular Therapies (LeJacq, New York), pp. 46–58.

Lewis, S. and L. Ryan.: 1986, 'The quality of community and the quality of life', Sociological Spectrum 6, pp. 397–410.

Lipowski, Z. J.: 1969, 'Psychological aspects of disease', Annals of Internal Medicine 71, pp. 1197–1206.

Lomas, J., L. Pickard and A. Mohide: 1987, 'Patient versus clinician item generation for quality-of-life measures: The case of language-disabled adults', Medical Care 25, pp. 764–769.

Mai, F. M., F. N. Mckenzie and W. J. Kostick: 1986. 'Psychiatric aspects of heart transplantation: Preoccupative evaluation and postoperative-sequelae', British Medical Journal 292, pp. 311–313.

McCullough, L. B.: 1984, 'The concept of quality of life: A philosophical analysis', in N. K. Wegner, M. E. Mattson, C. D. Furberg, and J. Elinson (eds.), Assessment Of Quality of life In Clinical Trials of Cardiovascular Therapies (LeJacq, New York), pp. 25–26.

McNeil, B., R. Weichselbaum and S. Pauker: 1981, 'Tradeoffs between quality and quantity of life in laryngeal cancer', Special Article Speech and Survival. New England Medical Journal 305, pp. 983–987.

Mayou, R: 1990. 'Quality of life in cardiovascular disease', Psychotherapy and Psychosomatics 54 pp. 99–109.

Mayou, R. A.: 1979, 'Course and determinants of reaction to myocardial infarction', British Journal of Psychiatry 134, pp. 588–594.

Mor, M. Z. Stalker, R. Scher, H. I. Scher, C. Cimma, D. Park, A. M. Flaherty, M. Kiss, P. Nelson, L. Laliberte, R. Schwartz, P. A. Marks and H. F. Oettigen: 1988, 'Day hospital as an alternative to inpatient cae for cancer patients: a random assignment trial', Journal of Clinical Epidemiology 41, p. 771.

Muthny, F. A., U. Koch and S. Stump: 1990, 'Quality of life in oncology patients', Psychotherapy and Psychosomatics 54, pp. 145–160.

Osaba, D.: 1991, Effect of Cancer On Quality of Life (CRC Press Inc., Baca Raton, Florida)

Osoba, D., N. K. Aranson and J. E. Till: 1991, 'A piratical guide for selecting quality-of-life measures in clinical tests and practice', in D. Osoba (ed.), Effect Of Cancer On Quality Of Life (CRC Press, Inc., Boca Raton, Florida).

Padella, G. V., C. Presant, V. M. Grant, G. Metter, J. Lipsett and E. Heidi: 1983, 'Quality of life index for patients with cancer', Research in Nursing and Health 6, pp. 117–125.

Parmenter, T. R.: 1988, 'An analysis of the dimensions of quality of life for people with physical disabilities', in R. I. Brown (ed.), Quality of Life For Handicapped People (Croom Helm, London), pp. 1–36.

Parmenter, T. R: 1992, 'Quality of life of people with developmental disabilities', International Review of Research in Mental Retardation 18, pp. 247–287.

Powell, V. and C. Powell: 1987, 'Quality of life measurement', Journal of Medical Ethics 123, pp. 222–223.

Raczynski, J. M. and A. Obermann: 1990, 'Cardiovascular surgery patients', in B. Spilker (ed.), Quality of Life Assessment In Clinical Trials (Raven Press, New York Press), pp. 295–322.

Richardson, J.: 1991, 'Economic assessment of health care: Theory and practice', Australian Economic Review, 1st quarter pp. 4–21.

Roessler, R. T.: 1990, 'A quality of life perspective on rehabilitation counselling', Rehabilitation Counselling Bulletin 34, pp. 82–90.

Rosenfield, S.: 1992, 'Factors contributing to the subjective quality of life of the chronic mentally ill', Journal of Health and Social Bebaviour 33, pp. 299–315.

Sage, W. M., M. H. Rosenthal and J. F. Silverman: 1986, 'Is intensive care worth it? An assessment of input and outcome for the critically ill', Cortical Care Medicine 14, p. 777.

Schalock, R. L.: 1991, The Concept Of Quality Of Life In The Lives Of Persons With Mental Retardation. Paper presented to 115th Annual Convention of the American Association on Mental Retardation, Washington, D.C.

Scherer, M. J.: 1988, 'Assistive disuse utilization and quality -of-life in adults with spinal cord injuries or cerebral palsy', Journal of Applied Rehabilitation Counselling 19, pp. 21–30.

Schipper, H., J. Clinch and V. Powell.: 1990, 'Definitions and conceptual issues', in B. Spilker (ed.), Quality of Life Assessments In Clinical Trials (Raven Press, New York), pp. 11–24.

Schipper, H., J. Clinch, A. McMurray and M. Levitt: 1984, 'Measuring the quality of life of cancer patients: The functional living index-cancer: Development and validation', Journal of Clinical Oncology 2, pp. 472–483.

Schoemaker, D., G. Burke, A. Dorr, R. Temple and M. A. Friedmann: 1990, 'A regulatory perspective', in B. Spilker (ed.), Quality of Life Assessment In Clinical Trials (Raven Press, New York), pp. 193–201.

Schumaker, S. A., R. T. Anderson and S. M. Czajkowski: 1990, 'Psychological tests and scales', in B. Spilker (ed.), Quality Of Life Assessments In Clinical Trials (Raven Press, New York), pp. 95–11.

Sexton, D. L. and B. H. Monro: 1988, 'Living with a chronic illness: The experience of women with chronic obstructive pulmonary disease (COPD)', Western Journal of Nursing Research 10, pp. 26–44.

Shapiro, P. A. and D. S. Kornfeld: 1989, 'Psychiatric outcome of heart transplant', General Hospital Psychiatry 11, pp. 352–357.

Siegrist, J. and A. Junge: 1990, 'Measuring the social dimension of subjective health in chronic illness', Psychotherapy and Psychosomatics 54, pp. 90–98.

Söder, M.: 1984, 'The mentaly retarded: Ideologies of care and surplus population' in L. Barton and S. Tomlinson (eds.), Special Education And Social Interests (Croom Helm, London).

Spilker, B.: 1990, 'Introduction', in B. Spiler (ed.), Quality Of Life Assessments In Clinical Trials (Raven Press, New York), pp. 3–9.

Spitzer, W. O., A. J. Dobson, J. Hall, E. Chestermann, J. Levi, R. Shepherd, R. N. Battista and B. R. Catehlove: 1981, 'Measuring the quality of life of cancer patients. A concise QL-Index for use by physicians', Journal of Chronic Disease 34, p. 585.

Stoddard, S.,: 1987, 'Independent living. Concepts and programs', American Rehabilitation 3, pp. 2–5.

Torrance , G. W.: 1986, 'Measurement of health state utilities for economic appraisal', Journal of Health Economics 5, pp. 1–30.

Torrance, G. W.: 1987, 'Utility approach to measuring health-related quality of life', Journal of Chronic Disease 40, pp. 593–600.

Till, J. E.: 1986, 'Quality-of-life assessment: beware the tyranny of the majority', Humane Medicine 2, p. 100.

Till, J. E.: 1991, 'Users (and some possible abuses) of quality-of-life measures', in D. Osoba (ed.), Effect Of Cancer On Quality Of Life (CRC Press Inc., Boca Raton, Florida) pp. 137–154.

Turner, R. R.: 1990, 'Rehabilitation', in B. Spilker (ed.), Quality of Life Assessments In Clinical Trials (Raven Press, New York), pp. 247–267.

Van Dam, F.: 1986, 'Quality of life: Methodological aspects', Cancer Bulletin (Paris) 73, pp. 607–613.

Vash, C. L.: 1984, 'Evaluation from the client's point of view', in A. S. Halpern and M. J. Fuhrer (eds.), Functional Assessment In Rehabilitation (Paul H. Brookes, Baltimore), pp. 2532–267.

von Nrewmann, J. and O. Morgenstern: 1947, Theory Of Games And Economic Behaviour (Princeton University Press, Princeton, N.J.).

Ware, J. E.: 1991, 'Measuring functioning, well-being, and other generic health concepts', in D. Osoba (ed.), Effects Of Cancer On Quality Of Life (CRS Press Inc., Boca Raton, Florida), pp. 8–23.

Ware, J. E.: 1984, 'Conceptualizing disease impact and treatment outcomes', Cancer 53, pp. 2316–2323.

Wegner, N. K., M. E. Mattson, C. D. Furberg and J. Elinson (eds.): 1984, 'Preface and overview: Assessment of quality of life in clinical trials of cardiovascular therapies, in N. K. Wegner, M. E. Mattson, C. D. Furberg and J. Elinson (eds.), Assessment Of Quality Of Lice In Clinical Trials Of Cardiovascular Therapies (LeJacq, New York), pp. 1–22.

Weinstein, M. C.: 1983, 'Cost-effective priorities for cancer prevention', Science 221, pp. 17–23.

Williams, A.: 1979, 'A note on "Trying to value life"', Journal of Public Economies 12, pp. 257–258.

Williams, A.: 1985, 'Economies of coronar artery bypass graftng', British Medical Journal 291, pp. 326–329.

Wood, P. H. N.: 1975, Classification Of Impairment And Handicap, Document WHO/ICDP/REV-CONF/75.15 (World Health Organization, Geneva).

World Health Organization: 1984, Constitution of World Health Organization, Basic Document (Author, Geneva).

World Health Organization: 1958, The First Ten Years Of The World Health Organization (Author, Geneva).

Young, R. F.: 1982, 'Marital adaption and response in chronic illness: The case of COPD' (Doctoral dissertation, Wayne State University) Dissertation Abstracts, 42: 4947A.

Zaner, R. M.: 1986, 'Soundings from uncertain places: Difficult pregnancies and imperiled infants', in P. R. Dokecki and R. M. Zaner (eds.), Ethics Of Dealing With Persons With Severe Handicaps (Paul H. Brookes, Baltimore).

Zubrad, C. G., M. Schneiderman and E. Frei et al.: 1960, 'Appraisal of methods for the study of chemotherapy of cancer in man: Comparative therapeutic trial of nitrogen mustard and triethylene thiophosphoramide', Journal of Chronic Disease 11, pp. 7–33.

School of Education,
Macquarie University,
2109 Sydney, NSW,
Australia.

DAVID R. EVANS

ENHANCING QUALITY OF LIFE IN

THE POPULATION AT LARGE

(Accepted 14 February, 1994)

ABSTRACT. The purpose of this review was to identify and discuss emerging issues in the literature on quality of life in the population at large. Interest in the topic has developed from a desire to compare cultural units, to develop normative data, and to establish programs to enhance quality of life. An attempt is made to impose some empirical and theoretical order on the numerous definitions and measures of quality of life, that have been used with the population at large. A taxonomy is provided that outlines the relationship among measures of quality of life. Following this discussion, studies identifying those factors that may influence quality of life in the population at large are examined, and a model linking these factors is proposed. The model includes Personal/Dispositional Factors, Biosociophysical Environmental Factors, General and Domain Specific Skills, Affective Tone, Social Support and Cognitive Appraisal as they relate to Quality of Life. Potential Quality of Life enhancement programs are considered with respect to their orientation (Person, Environment) and their mode of delivery (One on one, Education, Legislation). Recommendations concerning measures that can be implemented to enhance quality of life in the population at large are made.

Since the early 1940s there has been an increasing interest in the assessment of quality of life (Gross, 1966; Tolman, 1941). Sullivan (1992) stated that "quality of life" emerged as a political entity in the United States in the mid 1950s, and in Europe in the 1960s. The number of publications on quality of life was limited until the late 1970's, when the political entity finally became a scientific concern. Since then an exponential growth in the literature on quality of life has occurred in a broad range of disciplines, including psychology, medicine and sociology (Karlsson, 1992). Most of the literature in the past decade has been focused on the assessment of quality of life with specific populations, including cardiac patients (King *et al.*, 1992; Scheier *et al.*, 1989; Waltz and Badura, 1988), cancer patients (Chaturvedi, 1991; Chubon, 1987;

Social Indicators Research **33**: 47–88, 1994.

De Groot, 1986), the developmentally challenged (Kozleski and Sands, 1992; Ouellette-Kuntz, 1990), patients with fertility problems (Andrews *et al.*, 1991; Evans *et al.*, 1989; Hearn *et al.*, 1987a), psychiatric patients (Bigelow *et al.*, 1990; Chubon, 1987; Frisch *et al.*, 1992), and transplant patients (Grant *et al.*, 1990, O'Brien *et al.*, 1988). The suggested purpose for such assessments has been varied, including the evaluation of interventions, the selection and monitoring of patients for treatments, decision making concerning funding of procedures and programs, and drug trials (Cheng, 1988; Faden and Leplège, 1992; Fava, 1990; Goodinson and Singleton, 1989). Spilker *et al.* (1990) have compiled an extensive bibliograph of the literature on quality of life in a wide range of medical domains. In contrast, to the expanding interest in quality of life in such broad areas as medicine, developmental challenge, and gerontology, interest in quality of life in the population at large appears to have diminished over the past four decades. The focus of the present chapter is on the concept of quality of life as it relates to members of the population at large, between 18 and 65 years of age.

One of the main reasons for studying quality of life in the population at large was inherent in the social indicators movement (Evans *et al.*, 1985). In the late 1960's there was a recognition that something more than gross economic indicators such as the gross national product was required as a basis for comparing countries (Chubon, 1987). The alternative proposed was the social indicator, a measure reflecting not only the economic development, but also, the social development of a country (Johnston, 1988, Palys and Little, 1980). It quickly became obvious that while the social indicator provided information about a cultural unit (town, state, country), it provided little or no information about the quality of life of the specific individuals within the unit. This observation led to interest in the assessment of the subjective or perceived quality of life of population samples in such cultural units as the United States, Europe, and Australia (Andrews, 1991; Davis and Fine-Davis, 1991; Headey and Wearing, 1991). Interest in subjective indicators of quality of life has intensified as researchers have failed to find other than meagre, and often, inconsistent relationships between objective social indicators and subjective measures (Costa and McCrea, 1980; Davis and Fine-Davis, 1991). The concern of the social indicators movement continues to be comparison between cultural units, or within cultural units over time, whether objective or subjective measures of quality of life are used (Andrews, 1991; Davis and Fine-Davis, 1991).

Another reason for developing and evaluating quality of life measures in the general population has been to provide normative data against which to compare samples from specific populations. Often these data are collected in conjunction with the development of measures designed for use with the specific population, as a point of reference against which to compare individuals in the population of interest (Frisch *et al.*, 1992; McGee *et al.*, 1991; Pavot and Diener, 1993). Other measures have been designed to gather normative data on the population at large, and data on specific populations have been compared to this normative data as the standard of quality of life (Evans *et al.*, 1985; Grant *et al.*, 1990; Hearn *et al.*, 1987b). The latter approach seems to provide the most appropriate standard against which to gauge the success of procedures and programs directed toward special populations. That is, it enables an evaluation of a given intervention in the attainment of a normal level of quality of life in the recipients. In any event, the derivation of measures and normative data respecting the quality of life of the population as a whole is of interest in its own right.

A third reason for studying quality of life in the population at large is that it is the most apparent goal of health promotion activities directed toward the general public. Quality of life, which is frequently defined as subjective well-being, is considered by many to be synonymous with health as it was defined by the World Health Organization in 1947 (World Health Organization, 1947). Given the latter proposition, efforts directed toward health promotion require procedures that enhance quality of life. As the current reactive health care approach displays a diminishing ability to provide quality care at reasonable cost, policy analysts and government leaders have argued the importance of health promotion as a means to improve the quality of life of the population as a whole (Allan and Hall, 1988; Matarazzo, 1992, Tones, 1986, Williams *et al.*, 1991). In his presentation to the International Conference on Health Promotion on June 17, 1986 Epp (1986) as Minister of national Health and Welfare for Canada equated the new perspective on health to quality of life. Considerable emphasis has been placed on health promotion since the member states of the World Health Organization declared that their main social goal was "Health for All by the Year 2000" (Kickbusch, 1987). Sullivan (1991) the U.S. Secretary of Health and Human Services in releasing *Healthy People 2000*, a report detailing a health promotion program that took some four years to develop, stated that the first of three goals under the program was "... to increase the span of healthy life by preventing premature death, disability, and disease, and enhancing quality of life." (p. 293). Kaplan (1991) argues that the impact of health promotion programs will be measured in quality of life years. Clearly programs to enhance the quality of life of the general population and health promotion activities have the same measurable goal in the minds of many.

Despite a paucity of recent articles studying quality of life in the population at large, its study remains important in the continued development of social indicators, normative standards, and as the focal component of health promotion efforts. In the past twenty years, there have been many advances made in the understanding of quality of life in the general population. These developments will be discussed under the following headings: The many Definitions of Quality of Life; Factors Affecting Quality of Life; Toward a theory of Quality of Life; and Programs to Enhance Quality of Life. It is evident from the literature that much has been accomplished in the past two decades, however, it is equally evident that there is still considerable research to be done before effective programs that enhance quality of life become a reality. This paper should give the reader a sense of what has been accomplished, and what remains to be achieved.

THE MANY DEFINITIONS OF QUALITY OF LIFE

Romney *et al.* (1992) have noted the "... countless definitions of quality of life." (p. 166). Faden and Leplège (1992) observed that while quality of life has common sense appeal and meaning, there is little agreement among scholars concerning its definition. Chibnall and Tait (1990) were more direct, stating that quality of life is an elusive concept. As Mugenda *et al.* (1990) have pointed out, there is little consensus on the definition of quality of life, and therefore, little agreement on its measurement. What is evident from a review of the extensive literature of quality of life in the population at large is that to date no standard definition of quality of life has been adopted (King *et al.*, 1992; Sullivan, 1992). In the discussion that follows an attempt will be made to impose some order on the seeming confusion of terms and definitions.

The Empirical Relationship Among Measures of Quality of Life

Many authors use quality of life interchangeably with other concepts, such as well-being, psychological well-being, subjective well-being, happiness, life satisfaction, morale, positive and negative affect, the good life (Cheng, 1988; Diener, 1984; George, 1992; Rice, 1984). Others use quality of life as a higher order concept, which subsumes other concepts such as subjective well-being, life satisfaction, positive and/or negative affect (Davis and Fine-Davis, 1991; Frisch *et al.*, 1992; King *et al.*, 1992). Some authors still put psychological distress and psychological well-being on a continuum, despite numerous findings that oppose this proposition (Bech, 1990; Chibnall and Tait, 1990). Others argue that quality of life is a multidimensional concept, which is represented by multiple continua, such as life satisfaction, and positive and negative affect (Abbey and Andrews, 1986; Frisch *et al.*, 1992; Headey and Wearing, 1991; Pavot and Diener, 1993). A number of authors have observed, that despite the diversity of concepts often employed to represent and/or measure quality of life, there are high intercorrelations among the various constructs (Costa and McCrea, 1980; Faden and Leplège, 1992; George, 1992; Pavot and Diener, 1993; Pellizzari and Evans, 1991). Despite the 'countless' number of constructs that have been used to represent quality of life, there has been little effort to impose either empirical, or theoretical order upon them.

Pellizzari and Evans (1992) investigated the empirical relationships among a number of measures of quality of life. The sample was comprised of 212 introductory psychology students. The measures included the ten scales of the Quality of Life Questionnaire pertinent to students (Evans and Cope, 1989), a set of Perceived Quality of Life Scales designed for the study (Pellizzari, 1992), the Positive and Negative

Affect Schedule (Watson *et al.*, 1988), the Satisfaction with Life Scale (Diener *et al.*, 1985), and the Ryff Scales of Psychological Well-being (Ryff, 1989). The component scales were factor analyzed, and a one or two factor solution was deemed to best fit the data. The one factor solution, with 23 variables measuring quality of life at both global and specific levels, accounted for only 29.20% of variance among variables. The two factor solution accounted for 38.81% of the variance among variables. Neither of these solutions was promising in terms of identifying either a single common factor, or a more complex factor structure to describe the many definitions and measures of quality of life.

On the assumption that the factor analysis reported by Pellizzari and Evans (1992) was mixing global and component measures, the data were reanalyzed. When the global measures, the Quality of Life Score (Evans and Cope, 1989), the mean of the Perceived Quality of Life Scales, the Positive and Negative Affect scores, and the Satisfaction With Life score were factor analyzed a better solution was obtained. One factor was obtained, which accounted for 57% of the variance among variables, suggesting that they could be accounted for by a single definition. The correlations between each variable and the single factor were as follows: Perceived Quality of Life, 0.83; quality of Life Score, 0.83; Satisfaction With Life score, 0.77; Positive Affect score, 0.73; Negative Affect score, -0.59. Given the high loadings the factor can be identified as a global quality of life factor. This outcome starts to define empirically the relative relationship between various global measures of quality of life in a college sample. Studies with larger community based samples, and a variety of global and specific measures are required to further define the empirical relationship among the various measures that have been proposed as representative of quality of life.

In the absence of more definitive empirical studies an alternative is to try to identify a theoretical structure relating the various measures (Cheng, 1988; Groenland, 1990; Rice, 1984; Ryff, 1989). Cheng (1988), Groenland (1990), and Ryff (1989) have argued that much of the confusion in the definition of quality of life will remain until the theoretical relationship among measures is established. A first step is to identify a taxonomy or set of categories, under which to organize the definitions of quality of life. Rice (1984) and Groenland (1990) have suggested categories that might constitute a taxonomy of definitions of quality of life. Their efforts are a start, but a review of the literature on quality of life in the general population suggests that the taxonomies proposed to date require several more levels of categorization, and a rationale for the relationships among categories.

Toward a Taxonomy of Measures of Quality of Life

The first, and perhaps the most important, dichotomous category recognized by most, if not all, authors is that of objective vs. subjective measures of quality of life (Chubon, 1987; Evans *et al.*, 1985; Faden and Leplège, 1992; Groenland, 1990; King *et al.*, 1992). Objective measures, or social indicators, represent in a broad sense the individual's standard of living represented by verifiable conditions inherent in the given cultural unit (Allen, 1991; Evans *et al.*, 1985; Rice, 1984). The Quality of Life Index (Johnston, 1988) is an example of a measure of the objective aspect of quality of life. Perhaps, because low correlations have been found between objective and subjective measures, there are those authors, that have argued that quality of life is purely subjective (Chaturvedi, 1991; Cheng, 1988). Rice (1984) argued that high correlations between objective and subjective measures will only obtain when the objective criteria are important to those sampled, and the level of the given objective and perceived criteria match. Allen (1991) has proposed that to adequately measure quality of life, both objective and subjective measures must be employed in some combination.

Usually, subjective quality of life has been defined as the degree to which the individual's life is perceived to match some implicit or explicit internal standard or referent (Abbey and Andrews, 1987; Cheng, 1988, Jenkins, 1992, Pavot and Diener, 1993). Dimensions of comparison that have been suggested, include one's current and expected situation (Jenkins, 1992), actual functioning relative to aspirations (Chaturvedi, 1991), one's potential and one's achievements (Romney *et al.*, 1992), achieved goals and unmet needs (Brown, 1989, Frisch *et al.*, 1992), aspirations and achievements (Hughey and Bardo, 1987). However, it is possible to conceive of a subjective measure of quality of life in which the standard of comparison is an external referent. This is the model employed in most personality tests, in which the individual's responses are compared to those of a normative sample, or external referent. A number of authors have argued that measures of quality of life should rely less on self ratings based upon an internal referent, and more on a person's actual behaviour, and current conditions compared to external referents (Evans *et al.*, 1985; Jenkin, 1992; Matarazzo, 1992; Rice, 1984). The Quality of Life Questionnaire (Evans and Cope, 1989) was developed as a multidimensional measure using the rational-empirical approach to test construction. In this method the items comprising the measure are selected by item analysis of the responses of a normative sample. The subjective approach, which involves a normative sample, bases the value judgement about what represents a good quality of life on the values of the population sampled, not on the values of a single observer as in the social indicators method (Diener, 1984). Hence, within the subjective category of measures there are those that involve an external referent (normative data), and those that use an internal referent (a personal judgement).

For those measures that involve an internal referent there is some debate about whether the comparison that is made is to others, or to one's own goals, aspirations, potentials (Chubon, 1987; Diener, 1984; Pavot and Diener, 1993). That is, is the standard of comparison the self or others? There appears to have been little effort to develop measures that are based on such a social comparison model. However, given the extensive literature on social comparison in social psychology it seems that such an approach may have some promise. While Chubon (1987) raised the potential for such an approach to measurement, his measure, the Life Situation Survey (Chubon, 1987) is based on self comparisons, and not other oriented comparisons. To fit the social comparison model, words such as 'Compared to others my life is' would need to be included either in the instructions, or the items. Headey and Wearing (1988) use such a measure in their study to evaluate Sense of relative superiority as it relates to quality of life. As this distinction seems to have potential merit, and given the extensive literature on social comparison, it is included in the current taxonomy.

Another category that can be used to identify types of quality of life measures is the basis upon which the response is made. In the case of objective measures the basis is observation. For subjective measures having an external referent, and subjective measures that are internal referent, having a comparison based on others, the basis is cognitive. For those subjective measures that are internal referent, and have as the basis for judgement characteristics of the self, one other dimension has been proposed. Several authors have argued for a distinction between cognitive measures, namely life satisfaction, and affective measures of positive and negative affect (Abbey and Andrews, 1986; Groenland, 1990; Headey and Wearing, 1991; Pavot and Diener, 1993). Headey and Wearing (1991) ponder whether negative affect should be further subdivided into anxiety and depression. There is little support for this proposition at this time. There is good support for the distinction between cognitive and affective measures, and the further subdivision of affective measures into positive and negative dimensions.

The proposed taxonomy is shown in Table I, along with representative measures were they exist. It is evident that the majority of measures developed to date are in the life satisfaction domain, followed by the affective domain. One problem with such measures, that have an internal referent that relates to an individual standard, is that the standard can be changed quickly by the individual. Hence, when confronted with a stressful life event, individuals may change their aspirations, as a means of coping, thus changing the standard of comparison for the quality of life measure (Diener, 1984; Chaturvedi, 1991; Frisch et al., 1992). The latter argument may explain the findings that stressful life events have only a brief effect on quality of life. It is for this and other reasons that Jenkins (1992) and Matarazzo (1992), among others, have argued for improved and better standardized quality of life scales assessing specific behaviours. If one uses a subjective measure that is based on an external referent, and has associated norms based on the population at large, then the true effect of a stressful life event is more likely to be observed. As an example, an individual may well have a heart attack, and as a result change his or her aspirations, thus affecting the level of life satisfaction. If in this case a standardized measure, such as the Quality of Life Questionnaire (Evans and Cope, 1989) is used, then the impact of the heart attack can be gauged by comparison to a normative level of quality of life.

TABLE I

A Taxonomy of Quality of Life Measures

Method	Referent	Standard	Basis	Example Measure
Objective	External	Norms	Observation	QOL Index[1]
Subjective	External	Norms	Cognitive	QLQ[2]
	Internal	Others	Cognitive	
		Self	Cognitive	ESM[3]
				LSS[4]
				QOLI[5]
				QOLS[6]
				SWLS[7]
			Affective	ESM[3]
				PANAS[8]

[1] The Quality of Life Index (Johnston, 1988); [2] The Quality of Life Questionnaire (Evans and Cope, 1989); [3] The Event Sampling Method (Csikszentmihalyi and LeFevre, 1989); [4] The Life Situation Survey (Chubon, 1987); [5] The Quality of Life Inventory (Frisch *et al.*, 1992); [6] The Quality of Life Scale (Chibnall and Tait, 1990); [7] The Satisfaction With Life Scale (Diener *et al.*, 1985; Pavot and Diener, 1993); [8] The Positive And Negative Affect Scale (Watson *et al.*, 1988).

General Issues in the Measurement of Quality of Life

There are two other issues that transcend the categories included in the taxonomy. The first issue is the use of global versus domain specific measures. Most authors agree that quality of life as a whole is based upon an evaluation of one's life in a number of domains (Abbey and Andrews, 1987; Davis and Fine-Davis, 1991; Evans *et al.*, 1985; Groenland, 1990; McGee *et al.*, 1991). What is at issue is the derivation of the overall measure of quality of life from the evaluation of the constituent domains. Of concern is the management of the idiosyncratic nature of the various life domains, each having a different importance to each individual (Davis and Fine-Davis, 1991; Faden and Leplège, 1992; McGee *et al.*, 1991). One position can be referred to as the 'personal integrative model'. Under this model measures include only items related to 'life as a whole', thus requiring the individual to integrate the importance of each life domain into her or his response (Campbell *et al.*, 1976; Diener, 1984; Pavot and Diener, 1993). The Satisfaction With Life Scale (Diner *et al.*, 1985) is an example of a measure based upon the premise of this model. The opposite position is represented by the 'linear additive model'. Proponents of this model argue that overall quality of life is the sum of evaluations in each of a predetermined set of domains (Chibnall and Tait, 1990; Davis and Fine-Davis, 1991; Rice *et al.*, 1992). The Quality of Life Scale (Chibnall and Tait, 1990) is an example of a measure using the linear additive model. The remaining position is the 'weighted sum position'. To take care of the individual importance of each domain, the overall quality of life is calculated by summing the products of the individual's evaluation in each domain and the importance of each domain (Evans and Cope, 1989; Frisch *et al.*, 1992; McGee *et al.*, 1991). The Quality of Life questionnaire (Evans and Cope, 1989), the Quality of Life Inventory (Frisch *et al.*, 1992), and the Schedule for the Evaluation of Individual Quality of Life (McGee *et al.*, 1991) are all measures that base the overall measure of quality of life on a weighted sum of domain evaluations, taking into account the relative importance of each domain to the individual. Each uses a different method to accommodate individual differences in domain importance. Rice (1984) has suggested that efforts to take account of interaction, curvilinear, and differential weighting factors add little to the variance accounted for, when compared to the linear additive model. The issue of how to combine evaluations of life domains into an overall measure of quality of life requires further research, before a final model can be adopted.

The second issue concerns the stability of types of measure and/or domain measures over time (Chen, 1988; George, 1992; Goodinson and Singleton, 1989; Groenland, 1990). It is fair to say that the authors concerned with this issue have simply raised it as a consideration. There is little research directed toward defining which measures are trait, or state oriented. Cheng (1988) has argued that cognitive, and affective measures will exhibit differential levels depending on the time course of stressful life events. Goodinson and Singleton (1989) have suggested that domain based evaluations will vary over the life course. Groenland (1990) included in his taxonomy the need to categorize measures as being momentary, or structured, long term approaches. George (1992) has indicated that perhaps cognitive measures are more directed to the long term, while affect measures are sensitive to short term effects. The latter arguments suggest the need to consider distinguishing and/or developing trait and state measures of quality of life.

An attempt has been made in this section to impose some order on the many definitions and measures of quality of life. Overall measures of quality of life seem to have high correlations with each other; however, the theoretical relationship among them has yet to be established. The taxonomy that was developed should at least help researchers to be aware of the type of quality of life measure that is being used, and may perhaps provide a starting point for research that establishes the nature of the relationship among different conceptions of quality of life. Measures such as the quality of life year (Goodinson and Singleton, 1989; Kaplan, 1991; McCulloch, 1991), a measure of life expectancy adjusted for quality of life, are perhaps premature until there is some agreement on what is an appropriate measure of quality of life. There seem to be an ample number of cognitive and affective measures of perceived quality of life to choose from, but what is required are more measures based on external referents, having norms against which to compare individuals (Evans *et al.*, 1985; Jenkins, 1992; Matarazzo, 1992). Further, there is a need for more research into the method of integrating life domain evaluations into an overall measure, while taking into account individual differences. Finally, the issue of whether researchers need to consider a trait/state approach to the definition and measurement of quality of life needs attention.

FACTORS AFFECTING QUALITY OF LIFE

The purpose of this section is to examine research into factors that impact on quality of life. Notwithstanding the definitional problems noted in the previous section, the research reviewed will include studies using all definitions of quality of life, on the assumption that the measures are all highly correlated, and hence, may be considered as a whole. However, it is important to be aware, that some of the differential findings may be the result of what might be referred to as measurement variance. The rationale for identifying factors that influence quality of life is twofold; first they are the basis for developing a theory of quality of life, and second they provide the raw material for generating programs to enhance quality of life in the population at large. The studies reviewed fall into two easily identified dichotomies depending on whether single, or multiple factors are studies, and whether the studies are cross sectional or longitudinal in design. The studies will be discussed under the latter categories starting with single variable cross sectional studies, and ending with multiple variable longitudinal studies.

Cross Sectional Studies of Single Variables

Eight studies were identified that evaluated the relationship between specific variables and measures of quality of life in the population at large using a cross sectional design. The results of these studies are summarized in Table II. Several domain specific measures have been found to be related to quality of life: Marital satisfaction, Job satisfaction, Financial satisfaction, Community satisfaction, Marital adjustment, Religious satisfaction, Family life quality, and Family well-being. Two personality measures, self esteem and hardiness, and two communications measures, Intimacy and Expressiveness have been related to quality of life. A resource variable, Income, and an environmental variable, Urban vegetation were also related to quality of life. Although, there is no clear pattern among these results, they do suggest some of the variables that might be manipulated in an effort to enhance quality of life. Several of these authors have also looked at the relationship between other variables and domain specific measures of quality of life, for example Poloma and Pendleton (1990) report the relationship between a number of measures of Religious behaviour and Belief, and Religious satisfaction. However, they have not looked at the direct effects of these variables on quality of life. Nor have they investigated

TABLE II

Univariate relationships observed with quality of life in cross sectional studies

Author	Variable	Quality of Life Variable	Relationship
Evans et al. (1993c)	Self Esteem	Quality of Life	$r = 0.53$
	Hardiness	Quality of Life	$r = 0.41$
	Marital Satisfaction	Quality of Life	$r = 0.36$
	Intimacy	Quality of Life	$r = 0.72$
	Expressiveness	Quality of Life	$r = 0.59$
	Job Satisfaction	Quality of Life	$r = 0.51$
George (1992)	Financial Resources (Income)	Subjective Well-being	$r = 0.12–0.43$[1]
	Financial Satisfaction	Subjective Well-being	$r = 0.14–0.59$[2]
Hughey and Bardo (1987)	Community Satisfaction	Quality of Life	$R = 0.31$
Leslie and Anderson (1988)	Domestic Role (Husbands and Wives)	Subjective Well-being	non sig.
	Domestic Role	Marital Satisfaction	non sig.
Parasuraman et al. (1989)	Marital Adjustment	Quality of Life	$r = 0.41$
	Job Satisfaction	Quality of Life	$r = 0.52$
Poloma and Pendleton (1990)	Religious Satisfaction	Life Satisfaction	$r = 0.33$
Rettig et al. (1991)	Family Life Quality	Quality of Life	$r = 0.64$
	Global Family Well-being	Quality of Life	$r = 0.62$
Sheets and Manzer (1991)	Urban Vegetation	Quality of Life	sig. effect

[1] Number of studies = 20, [2] Number of studies = 14

the indirect effects of these variables on quality of life (i.e., through other variables).

Cross Sectional Studies Involving Multiple Variables

This group of studies falls into three categories. First, there are those, in which a multiple correlation approach has been used to investigate the relationship and interrelationships between a number of variables, and quality of life in the population at large. In the second group of studies, multiple correlation methods have been used in a path analysis to evaluate a predetermined model of relationships among variables. Third, there are a set of studies that have used path analytic methods to evaluate several models to determine the best model of quality of life. There are two popular models that have been proposed to explain the relationship between quality of life and other variables; the top-down model, and the bottom-up model (Diener, 1984; Headey *et al.*, 1991; Lance *et al.*, 1989). The top-down model is based on the premise that quality of life is an enduring characteristic that causes certain outcomes in the individual's life. In contrast, the bottom-up model rests on the proposition that particular variables influence and individual's quality of life. In that these models are causal in nature it is difficult to test them in a cross sectional study. Lance *et al.* (1989) have detailed the assumptions that must be met in order to evaluate causality in a cross sectional study.

There are a considerable number of studies that have as their focus, the quality of working life, and Loscocco and Roschelle (1991) have provided a partial review of this area. The majority of the latter studies were excluded from current consideration, because they did not extend to overall quality of life in the general population. Parasuraman *et al.* (1989) studied the impact of wives 'employment on the husbands' quality of life, while evaluating the effect of demographic variables, the husbands' time commitment to work, and the husbands' evaluation of work-family conflict. For the relationship between wife's employment status and the husband's quality of life, the multiple correlation was 0.14. When the control or demographic variables were entered alone, and along with the husband's time commitment to work, the multiple correlation did not change significantly. When the husband's evaluation of work-family conflict was added as a final step the multiple correlation jumped to 0.50, and the regression coefficients for wife's employment status and the husband's evaluation of work-family conflict were significant. Keller (1987) studied the relationship between demographic variables, including gender and race, work variables, and non-work variables on quality of life. He obtained an adjusted multiple correlation of 0.56 between these variables and quality of life. However, significant regression coefficients were obtained for only job satisfaction (0.13), home stress (-0.40), self esteem (0.24), and job level (0.18). Coefficients for job stress, education, age, sex, marital status, and race were not significant.

A sample of 162 dairy farm couples from Utah were studied by Ackerman *et al.* (1991) to identify which domains were related to global quality of life. Stepwise regression analyses were performed, for husbands and wives, to identify those domains, with or without the farm work domain, that are related to global quality of life. For husbands, satisfaction with farm work, self, health and finances had a multiple correlation of 0.59 with global quality of life. When satisfaction with farm work was excluded from the analysis, satisfaction with self, leisure, health, and finances entered the equation, and a multiple correlation of 0.53 was observed. In the case of the wives, satisfaction with leisure, farm work, self, family, finances, and house entered the equation, and the multiple correlation with global quality of life was 0.53. When satisfaction with farm work was excluded from consideration, satisfaction with leisure, self, family, finances, and health entered the equation, and the multiple correlation was 0.48.

Woodruff and Conway (1992a) studied the impact of a set of health and fitness behaviours on quality of life in a sample of 5,082 randomly selected personnel in the U.S. Navy. To evaluate the stability of their findings Woodruff and Conway (1992a) used a random sampling procedure to split their sample in half. Then, they performed a hierarchical regression analysis to examine the relative contribution to quality of life of health and fitness status variables alone, and in conjunction with health and fitness behaviours. For the relationship between the health and fitness status variables and quality of life they obtained a multiple correlation of 0.40 and 0.43 for each sample, and the regression coefficients for health status (0.11, 0.15), fitness status (0.13, 0.19), and physical symptoms (-0.18, -0.14) were significant. When the health and fitness behaviours were added the multiple correlation increased to 0.52 and 0.49 respectively, and the regression coefficients for traffic risk (-0.09, -0.08), and accident control (0.25, 0.19) were significant. Addition of the health and fitness behaviour variables made a significant difference in the relationship among these variables and quality of life.

Evans *et al.* (1993b) studied the relationship between coping skills, social support and personality traits, and psychological well-being in a sample of individuals in the community, whose acute leukemia was in remission. When a step-wise multiple regression of the coping and social support variables on psychological well-being was performed the multiple correlation did not reach significance. When a similar analysis was carried out using personality variables, a multiple correlation of 0.80 was obtained with the personality dimensions, endurance (0.49), affiliation (0.57), cognitive structure (0.44), autonomy (0.35), and nurturance (-0.29). This study is included here as an example of the considerable literature that is beginning to compare the relationship between events and their management (bottom-up theories), and quality of life on the one hand, and the relationship between dispositions (top-down theories) and quality of life on the other hand. The complex of personality variables is comparable to what others have referred to as dispositional optimism (Scheier *et al.*, 1989).

Young (1991) carried out a study, that compared recently arrived and long term Canadians, and Salvadorian Refugees. The 60 recently arrived Salvadorian refugees completed a migration life events scale, measures of locus of control and self esteem, and the Quality of Life Questionnaire (Evans and Cope, 1989). Locus of control was found to moderate the effect of migration life events on quality of life. Refugees with a high number of migration life events, and an internal locus of control had a higher quality of life than those with an external locus of control. Similarly, self esteem was found to moderate the relationship between migration life events and quality of life. As might be expected, those refugees confronted with a large number of life events, having a high self esteem, had higher quality of life than those with lower self esteem. These findings provide further support for the role of personality variables in moderating the effect of stressful events on quality of life.

In a path analytic study Berry and Williams (1981) assessed the relationship between a number of factors, including quality of life, marital satisfaction, and income satisfaction. They studied a random sample of husbands and wives from Indiana, drawn in equal numbers from a metropolitan, and a nonmetropolitan area of the state. For the most part they obtained similar results for husbands and wives. They found that a number of dynamic processing, Economic and Noneconomic variables had direct relationships with quality of life, while others had indirect relationships through Agreement over family finances and/or Marital satisfaction, and Income satisfaction. Agreement over family finances had an indirect effect through Marital satisfaction and Income satisfaction. For wives and husbands the direct relationship between Marital satisfaction and quality of life was 0.47 and 0.35 respectively, and for Income satisfaction it was 0.20 and 0.42 respectively. Mugenda *et al.* (1990) used path analysis to investigate the relationships among demographic, financial, skill, and satisfaction measures, and quality of life. They interviewed 123 money managers from a sample of households in Iowa, two thirds of whom were women. Several demographic and financial variables, including Household size, and Current years savings had both direct and indirect relationships with quality of life. Others and only indirect relationship through such variables as Communication, Money management practices, and Satisfaction with financial status. communication, in turn, had an indirect relationship through Money management practices, which had an indirect relationship through Satisfaction with financial status. Direct relationships with quality of life were as follows: Household Size, 0.41; Marital status, 0.21; Sex, -0.15; Income, 0.44; Current years savings, -0.31; and Satisfaction with financial status, 0.37. Interestingly, Current years savings had a negative relationship with quality of life.

Headey and Wearing (1988) analyzed the responses of 584 participants in the third wave of the Australian Quality of Life panel study using a path analytic approach. They found that both Sense of relative superiority, and social network had direct and indirect relationships with quality of life. Indirect relationships were through Self esteem and Personal competence, each of which in turn had direct relationships with quality of life. Direct relationships with quality of life were as follows: Sense of relative superiority, 0.17; Social network, 0.18; Self esteem, 0.23; and Personal competence, 0.20. This study suggests the importance of social and personality variables to quality of life.

In a study with a random sample of 137 persons over 60, Russell (1990) investigated the interrelationships among demographic, recreation, and quality of life variables, using a path analysis. The results are included here, because if they were replicated in the population at large they would identify variables important in recreation and quality of life. Russell (1990) found that Sex and Education had an indirect relationship through Recreation participation, and Age had an indirect relationship through both Recreation Participation and Recreation satisfaction with quality of life. Recreation participation had an indirect relationship through Recreation satisfaction, which had a direct relationship with quality of life of 0.31.

Two studies were identified, that have been carried out to evaluate the top-down and/or bottom-up models of quality of life, using path analytic procedures with cross sectional data. Rice et al. (1992), in a study using a household sample of 823 persons, found that Work-family conflict had an indirect relationship with quality of life through Family satisfaction, Job satisfaction, and Leisure satisfaction, each of which had direct relationships with quality of life (0.43, 0.34, 0.18 respectively). Work-leisure conflict was found to have an indirect relationship through Job satisfaction and Leisure satisfaction. Rice et al. (1992) concluded that their results suggested support for an additive model of quality of life, in which quality of life in each domain combines to determine the overall quality of life. The latter is a bottom-up theory of quality of life. The second study by Lance et al. (1989) was carried out with 134 professors at the University of Georgia, who were from a random sample of 170 selected to participate. These authors argue that their data meet the assumptions for using cross sectional data to evaluate causal relationships. They tested the top-down, bottom-up, and bidirectional models of quality of life. In the bidirectional path analysis they found that the relationships with quality of life were as follows: Job satisfaction was bidirectional; Satisfaction with social activities was top-down;

and Marital satisfaction was bottom-up. They reported the following correlations with quality of life: Job satisfaction, 0.58; Satisfaction with social activities, 0.62; and Marital satisfaction, 0.51. While these two studies are suggestive of the causal relationships between the variables studied and quality of life they need to be replicated with a longitudinal sample.

Taken together these studies suggest both the range of variables contributing to quality of life, and the complexity of the interrelationships among them. A number of personality factors, such as, self esteem, endurance, and locus of control, appear to have a direct effect on quality of life, and also, tend to moderate the effects of the environment on the individual's quality of life. Several components in the individual's biological and social environment, such as, work-family conflict, employment status and level, agreement over family finances, and health and fitness status, have an impact on an individual's quality of life. Financial skills, and the practice of health and fitness behaviours, and participation in recreational activities, all appear to influence the individual's quality of life. Further, the availability of a social network seems to be important to an individual's quality of life. At a more complex level factors within specific life domains affect satisfaction in the particular domain, and in turn the individual's quality of life is affected. The results of these studies suggest some useful parts in the puzzle depicting the factors that influence quality of life, and the complexity of their interrelationships.

Longitudinal Studies of Single Variables

As might be expected the majority of longitudinal studies deal with multiple variables. However, there are a number of studies that can be considered to deal with single variables in that they deal with changes in variables over time, and use correlational or univariate methods of analysis. They study of changes in the effect of race on quality of life by Thomas and Hughes (1986) can be considered to fall into this category. Using data from the General Social Survey in the U.S. for the years 1972 to 1985 (excepting 1979 and 1981) they compared 'blacks' and 'whites' on six measures of quality of life. They concluded, that despite changes in civil rights just prior to the study period, whites experienced better quality of life than blacks. The differential was constant over the years sampled. For both groups, Life satisfaction, Marital happiness, and Trust in people, showed a significant decline, and Anomie showed a significant increase over the years studied. Thomas and Hughes (1986) advanced three explanations to account for the lack of a change due to the effect of the civil rights legislation.

Latten (1989) used a combination of cross sectional and longitudinal techniques to explore whether an individual's life course, the result of biological aging, affected quality of life. Using data gathered in the Quality of Life Surveys for 1974, 1977, 1980, and 1983 in the Netherlands from some 3,000 respondents 18 years and older, Lattan (1989) examined the effects of the period in which participants lived, their birth generation, and life course on quality of life. Support was found for a general life course in quality of life regardless of birth generation and period. What was observed was relative stability to age 30 followed by a decline until about age 56, at which time an incline starts. Latten (1989) suggested that despite an increase in negative life events after age 56 acceptance of old age causes the increase in quality of life after that age.

In a study of 4942 persons in the U. S. whose original data were collected between 1971 and 1975, and follow up data between 1981 and 1984, Costa et al. (1987) found considerable stability in quality of life over time. In short they found that future quality of life was best predicted by past quality of life rather than demographic variables, such as marital status, race, sex and age. Further, they observed that changes in marriage, work, and residence had little impact on quality of life at least over a decade. They concluded that "environmental effects on subjective well-being appear to be limited in magnitude, duration, and scope. At any given time, well-being scores appear to be better predicted by earlier scores than by objective circumstances, even when circumstances have been altered dramatically since earlier scores were obtained" (Costa et al., 1987, p. 305).

Brandtstädter and Baltes-Götz (1990) studied 1228 participants (married couples) from an urban area in southwestern Germany who were found to be representative of the general population. Data were gathered in 1983, 1985, and 1987. Among other things, they examined correlations among variables for the 1983, and 1987 data. Personal control, and Autonomous control, and Heteronomous control over development were all correlated with quality of life and marital adjustment on both occasions. They concluded from these findings that persons scoring high on either Personal, or Autonomous control over development had higher quality of life and marital adjustment. In contrast, those high on Heteronomous control over development had lower quality of life, and marital adjustment. Personal and Autonomous control over development seem similar to internal Locus of control, and Heteronomous control over development seems similar to external Locus of control. They also explored the relationships between changes in these variables between 1983 and 1987. Increases in Personal and Autonomous control over development were associated with increases in quality of life, whereas increases in Heteronomous control over development were associated with decreases in quality of life.

This group of studies begin to identify some of the factors that influence an individual's quality of life over time. All of the studies suggest that an individual's quality of life remains relatively stable over time. This stability is maintained despite the impact of a variety of life events, that seem to have only a brief transitory effect. Legislation designed to improve the social environment of blacks in the United States seemed to have little relative effect on their quality of life in the thirteen years following its passage. Changes in the personality variable, locus of control, over time did appear to produce improvement in the quality of life of individuals. This set of studies adds some important information, upon which to base a model of those factors that influence quality of life, and which might be important to consider in developing programs to enhance quality of life in the population at large.

Longitudinal Studies Involving Multiple Variables

These studies can be grouped under the same methods as used in the section on cross sectional studies involving multiple variables. Using a sample of 519 U. S. Navy personnel, Woodruff and Conway (1992b) investigated the effect of changes in health/fitness status, and health behaviours on quality of life. The participants completed questionnaires in 1986, 1987, and 1988, and residualized gain scores were computed for each variable for the period 1986–1987, and 1987–1988. A multiple correlation of 0.21 and 0.30 was obtained between Health/Fitness status and quality of life for the two periods respectively. When changes in the Health behaviours were added into the regression, multiple correlations of 0.27 and 0.33 were calculated, and the change in the amount of variance accounted for in each period was significant. Accident control had a significant regression coefficient for both periods, and Wellness maintenance and enhancement had a significant regression coefficient for the first period only. Increases in health/fitness status resulted in increases in quality of life, and increases in health protective behaviours increased quality of life independently of the individual's health/fitness status.

Hoopes and Lounsbury (1989) investigated the impact of a vacation, on various domains of quality of life, and overall quality of life. They surveyed 168 working adults one to two weeks prior to their vacation, and one week after their vacation, 129 participated on both occasions. In separate hierarchical regression analyses prevacation measures were entered first followed by vacation measures, and in each case the postvacation measure was the dependent measure. In each case the premeasure had a high multiple correlation with the post measure. For satisfaction with each of leisure, marriage/family, nature, and work while on vacation, the increment in the variance accounted for was significant. As with the latter domains satisfaction with the vacation resulted in a significant increase in the variance accounted for by prevacation quality of life. Vacation satisfaction was found to produce an increase in overall quality of life.

In a longitudinal study using data from the Australian Quality of Life panel study, Headey and Wearing (1990) investigated the impact of methods of coping with critical life events in three areas. The life event areas were financial and job; health; and personal relationships. Path analyses in each area were carried out for 78, 72, and 128 subjects respectively. Data collected in 1983 and 1985 were analyzed. Participants responded to life events and coping inventories in the 1985 survey concerning the two year intervening period. The measure of quality of life was negative affect, for which, 1983 and 1985 data were available. For all categories of events 1983 quality of life, instrumental events, and avoidance coping had significant path coefficients with 1985 quality of life. In each case instrumental coping was found to reduce negative affect, and avoidance coping increased negative affect. The findings suggest both a dispositional component in that as 1983 quality of life increased so 1985 quality of life increased, and a skill based factor, in that instrumental coping with prior events increased 1985 quality of life, and avoidant coping decreased it.

Costa and McCrae (1980) obtained data for 234 men who were mailed quality of life questionnaires every 3 months for a year. In the third mailing they included personality measures. From the 16 PF short form data a neuroticism and an extraversion score were calculated. The neuroticism and extraversion scores were also available from the Eysenck Personality Inventory. For most analyses the extraversion scores were significantly related to positive affect and overall quality of life, while neuroticism was related to negative affect on all four occasions. They proposed a model to account for the correlations, suggesting that extraversion has an indirect effect on overall quality of life through positive affect, and neuroticism has an indirect effect on quality of life through negative affect.

Brief *et al.* (1993) derived a model that integrates top-down and bottom-up models of quality of life. They argued that personality dispositions, and objective life circumstances influence an individual's interpretation of circumstances, which in turn influence quality of life. They studied participants in three waves of the Second Duke Longitudinal Study, with data collected every two years between 1970 and 1976. A path analysis was carried out on the data for 336 participants to evaluate the proposed model longitudinally. Measures of Negative affectivity and Objective health were included from the first wave, the measure of interpretation of health was taken from the second wave, and the quality of life measure was taken from the third wave. They found that Personality (Negative affectivity) and Objective life circumstances (Actual health) each had an indirect effect on quality of life through the Interpretation of Life Circumstances (self-rated health). Interpretation of life circumstances had a direct effect on quality of life. They also did cross sectional analyses on the data for each wave, for which the results were identical to those for the longitudinal study.

The studies reviewed in this section reveal a myriad of relationships between a vast array of variables and quality of life. What is more evident is the complexity of the relationship among variables as they relate to, or influence quality of life. Efforts to develop and test several models of quality of life are also evident. Generally, three categories of variables seem to be related to, or influence an individual's quality of life: quality of life in a range of life domains; personality variables; and skill variables, such as coping skills, communication skills, and money management skills. In the next section, an effort will be made to derive a model to account for these relationships, with due regard for the models that have already been proposed and tested. It is imperative that models be developed to drive future research, such that effective interventions can be developed to enhance quality of life in the population at large (Allen, 1991; Diener, 1984).

TOWARD A THEORY OF QUALITY OF LIFE

A review of the research on factors affecting quality of life, suggests that there are a number of dimensions that must be considered when constructing a theoretical model of quality of life. The first dimension of note is satisfaction, whether it be life satisfaction, or a domain specific satisfaction, such as job satisfaction, family satisfaction, or leisure satisfaction. Satisfaction is in essence what Lazarus (1991) has referred to as cognitive appraisal. He defines appraisal as an evaluation of what is believed about the significance of what is happening for one's general or specific well-being, or quality of life. The second dimension has to do with skills, which can be subdivided into general and specific skills. General or generic skills (Cowen, 1991), for example communication skills, problem solving skills, and so forth, can be considered important in most if not all life domains. On the other hand specific skills are relevant to a particular domain, such as money management skills and the financial domain (Mugenda et al., 1990), sexual skills and the partner or marital domain (Andrews et al., 1991). A third dimension that has been explored by some authors, and seems important to include in any model is social support (Abbey and Andrews, 1986; Headey and Wearing, 1988). A forth dimension that has received considerable attention is the impact of personality or dispositional factors on quality of life (Costa et al., 1987; Diener, 1984; Evans et al., 1993b). The fifth, and final dimension includes a range of biosociophysical environmental factors that have been found to impact on quality of life (Allen, 1991; Headey and Wearing, 1991; Loscocco and Roschelle, 1991). Stokols (1992) has provided an extensive list of many of the sociophysical environmental factors that can be included in this dimension, which in addition to critical life events (Headey and Wearing, 1990), and significant medical events (Scheier et al., 1989) makes up an extensive set of events or conditions in the biological, social, and physical environment that may affect an individual's quality of life. Figure 1 depicts a model that shows the potential interactions between these five dimensions in determining an individuals quality of life at any point in time. It is envisaged that the model can be applied equally well to overall life quality or life quality in a specific domain. The proposed relationships are based on an integration of the findings reviewed above, and the several efforts by others to develop, or test specific theories (Brief et al., 1993; Diener, 1984; Headey and Wearing, 1989; Lance et al., 1989).

The proposed relationships shown in the model in figure 1 are influenced by a number of current theories. First, Headey and Wearing (1989, 1991) have proposed a dynamic equilibrium theory, which involves three components. They hold that as long as the individual's environmental events/conditions remain stable, then quality of life will remain stable, because of the influence of stable personality/dispositional characteristics. However, when the individual's environmental events/conditions deviate from the normal stable pattern, then quality of life will be influenced. The impact of environmental events/conditions that deviate from the norm is only temporary, because personality traits influence the response to the events/conditions, and a return to stability. Second, another influence is provided by those authors that have argued the importance of environmental conditions in determining an individual's quality of life (Allen, 1991; Stokols, 1992). Third, Lance et al. (1989) proposed that the relationship between

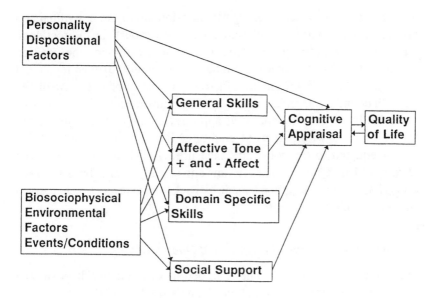

Fig. 1. A model of factors affecting quality of life.

cognitive appraisals of life quality and quality of life is bidirectional, rather than either top-down, or bottom-up. Fourth, Brief *et al.* (1993) have provided a theory that suggests that the impact of personality/ dispositional and environmental factors on quality of life is mediated through cognitive appraisal of life quality.

Cognitive Appraisal and Quality of Life

What has been referred to as either life satisfaction, or specific domain satisfaction (job satisfaction, marital satisfaction, financial satisfaction) can be viewed as a cognitive appraisal in the sense used by Lazarus (Lazarus, 1991; Lazarus and Folkman, 1984). It is proposed that cognitive appraisal of life in general, or of specific domains has a reciprocal relationship with quality of life. That is the relationship follows the bidirectional model that has been proposed and supported by a number of authors (Headey *et al.*, 1991; Lance *et al.*, 1989). It could be that depending on the salience of a particular domain to the individual at a particular point in time the relationship might variously be bidirectional, top-down, or bottom-up. Finally, it is argued, following the position of Brief *et al.* (1993), that the impact of personality/dispositional, and biosociophysical environmental factors on quality of life is mediated through cognitive appraisal of one's life circumstances. These propositions would suggest that cognitive appraisal of one's life circumstances can be equated with perceived quality of life, and that quality of life is best equated to the constructs measure by such instruments as the Quality of Life Questionnaire (Evans and Cope, 1989). The latter position is based on the arguments made by Rice (1984) respecting perceived and objective quality of life.

Personality/Dispositional Factors and Quality of Life

There are those authors who have argued that personality/dispositional factors are the only determinants of one's quality of life (Costa and McCrae, 1980; Costa *et al.*, 1987). Costa and McCrae (1980) postulated that particular personality traits impact upon either positive, or negative affect to determine an individual's cognitive appraisal of life circumstances. A number of personality/dispositional factors have been found to be related to, and/or to influence the cognitive appraisal of an individual's life circumstances: Dispositional optimism (Scheier *et al.*, 1989); A complex of PRF-E dimensions of personality (Evans *et al.*, 1993b; Self esteem (Evans *et al.*, 1993c; Headey and Wearing, 1988, Young, 1991); Hardiness (Evans *et al.*, 1993c); Internal/external locus of control (Abbey and Andrews, 1987; Brandtstädter, and Baltes-Götz, 1990; Young, 1991). The majority of authors do not hold the extreme position of Costa and McCrae (1980), rather they acknowledge that environmental factors under certain circumstances also influence an individual's cognitive appraisal of life circumstances (Abbey and Andrews, 1986; Headey and Wearing, 1989; 1991; Loscocco and Roschelle, 1991; Scheier *et al.*, 1989).

Biosociophysical Environmental Factors; Events/Conditions

The term conditions is used to refer to a steady state within the individual's biological, social, or physical environment. It is recognized that certain conditions in the individual's environment may impact on the appraisal of life circumstances, examples are poverty/wealth, genetic risk/health factors, polluted/clean air. A number of these conditions are routinely evaluated in measures of social indicators, such as the Quality of Life Index (Johnston, 1988). On the other hand, events in the proposed model refer to major changes in the biosociophysical environment. Examples are a myocardial infarction, loss of one's job, or a flood. The impact of environmental conditions and events on an individual's cognitive appraisal of life circumstances has been postulated to be moderated by such factors as the skills (general and specific) one has (Cocking, 1992; Csikszentmihalyi, 1990; Csikszentmihalyi and LeFevre, 1989; Headey and Wearing, 1990), the social support available (Abbey and Andrews, 1986; Brief and Atieh, 1987; Headey and Wearing, 1988), and the affective tone produced by the condition/event (Headey and Wearing, 1989). There is empirical support for many of these effects. Several authors have postulated that personality/dispositional factors have an impact on the individual's skills, affective tone, and social support (Diener, 1984; Bigelow *et al.*, 1990; Scheier *et al.*, 1989, Lazarus, 1993). It should be noted that the direction of the relationship between all of the variables in the model is most likely bidirectional. For example, self esteem will affect the spirit with which the individual copes with an environmental condition/event, and in turn the outcome of dealing with an environmental condition/event will affect self esteem (Diener, 1984).

PROGRAMS TO ENHANCE QUALITY OF LIFE

For the purpose of the present discussion, health promotion, and programs to enhance quality of life are taken to have the same goal (Sullivan, 1991). To date there have been few if any efforts to develop interventions directed toward the enhancement of quality of life *per se* (Frisch, 1992). Programs to enhance quality of life can be considered under two major categories: the orientation of the program; and the mode of program delivery. Programs can have one of two orientations; they can be directed toward the person, or the environment (Castillo-Salgado, 1984, Evans *et al.*, 1985; Stokols, 1992). Stokols (1992) has suggested that person oriented programs can be directed toward biogenetic, psychological, and behavioral aspects, while environment focused programs can be directed towards geographic, archeological, technological, and sociocultural factors. The mode of program delivery might be to develop individual based programs, educational programs, to foster social action and/or government change. With the factors that affect quality of life in mind, and the orientation of programs and the mode of program delivery as categories, potential programs will be considered in what follows.

ORIENTATION OF QUALITY OF LIFE ENHANCEMENT PROGRAMS

Person Oriented Programs

As more and more studies demonstrate the importance of stable personality characteristics as determinants of perceived quality of life the need to consider programs to engender and/or modify dispositions gains momentum (Evans *et al.*, 1993b, c; Sullivan, 1991; WHO Regional Office for Europe, 1986a). It is obvious that many of the personality traits or dispositions that individual's develop are established in childhood, hence, programs to encourage appropriate dispositions in childhood are essential (Brandtstädter and Baltes-Götz, 1990; Cowen, 1991; Lazarus, 1993). There are also programs, designed to modify self esteem, locus of control, and hardiness, available for adults (Frey and Carlock, 1989, 1991). One other disposition that may be important is the "culture of character" suggested by Sullivan (1991). By this she means "... a way of thinking, being, and acting that promotes responsible behaviour, and the adoption of life styles that are maximally conducive to good health" (p. 293–294).

The other major domain of person oriented programs, that are potentially important in enhancement programs, are those directed toward the skills of the individual, whether they are general in nature, and hence, tenable in all aspects of life, or they are appropriate to a single domain (WHO Regional Office for Europe, 1986a). Cowen (1991) suggested the following as generic skills: interpersonal skills; communication skills; problem solving skills; assertiveness, and skills directed toward emotional control. Others have also identified important general skills, for which there are already programs, such as communications skills (Evans *et al.*, 1993a), problem solving, and shared problem solving skills (Berry and Williams, 1987; Evans *et al.*, 1981, Kickbusch, 1987) Several authors have noted the importance of coping skills in enhancing quality of life (Epp, 1986, Evans *et al.*, 1989; Lazarus, 1993), and there are a number of programs directed toward developing such skills. Two modes of coping that have long been recognized as important are those identified by Brandtstädter and Baltes-Götz (1990) as assimilative and accommodative coping. Assimilative coping is appropriate when the individual can modify the environmental condition or event. When the latter is not possible, then the individual must use accommodative coping and modify her or his goals, aspirations, and so forth (Headey *et al.*, 1991; Cheng, 1988; Csikszentmihalyi and LeFevre, 1989). In that both these modes of coping will result in enhanced cognitive appraisals of life circumstances, both are important in programs designed to enhance quality of life. Other modes of coping that are important at other stages of dealing with environmental conditions and events are those directed at the perception of stress or affective tone, such as the ability to relax, meditation and exercise (Evans *et al.*, 1989). There have been few studies directed toward identifying domain specific skills that might be included in enhancement programs, but to date a few have been identified in the financial domain (Berry and Williams, 1987; Mugenda *et al.*, 1990), and the marital domain (Andrews *et al.*, 1991; Berry and Williams, 1987).

Another person oriented approach is to enhance the individual's social support network (Benum and Anstrop, 1987; Epp, 1986; WHO Regional Office for Europe, 1986a). There is an extensive literature on social support, and its review was beyond the scope of the present paper. There are no doubt programs in the social support area, as in other specific areas touched upon in this paper, that could be implemented and evaluated in programs to enhance quality of life. Benum and

Anstrop (1987) evaluated the impact of a network stimulation program for middle aged woman in a new satellite town near Oslo. Of the 50 women in the enhancement program 26 participated in a variety of group activities, porcelain painting, exercise, and social activity. Compared to a nonintervention control group of 50 women, the participants in the program were found to have improved their social networks, and to have increased quality of life and self esteem, a year after the program was initiated. Those who did not participate did not profit from the program. Social networks may also be facilitated by programs directed toward changes in the social environment.

Environment Oriented Programs

There are a number of authors, who have advocated the development of programs to enhance quality of life by changing aspects of the biological, social, or physical environment (Cocking, 1992; Epp, 1986; Loscocco and Roschelle, 1991; WHO Regional Office for Europe, 1986a). Such programs may be global in nature (e.g., improvement of air quality), or specific to particular environments (e.g., work, home). Tones (1986) has suggested that social engineering programs may be required to modify social environments, and hence, enhance quality of life. Stokols (1992) has listed a number of health promotion programs directed toward enhancing quality of life, by modifying factors in the biosociophysical environment (see Stokols, 1992, Table IV, p. 15). Some of the programs, he has suggested have been implemented, but as is often the case, their impact on quality of life has not been evaluated.

MODE OF QUALITY OF LIFE ENHANCEMENT PROGRAM DELIVERY

Intervention with Individual Clients

It follows from the current health (illness) system that one mode of health promotion is in the physicians's or the psychologist's office with individual clients (Allen, 1991; Castillo-Salgado, 1984). Their are other professionals, including lawyers, financial consultants, and insurance brokers, who also work with individual clients in this manner. Evans

(1993; Evans *et al.*, 1993c) has suggested that the Quality of Life Questionnaire (Evans and Cope, 1993) can be used to review the quality of each of the life domains of an individual on an annual basis ("Have you had your annual psychological checkup?"). Once reviewed the individual can be provided counselling, advised of programs in specific domains, and given training in generic/specific skills as required. A program such as this was implemented at the Pioneer Health Centre in St. Mary's Road, Peckham, England in 1935 (Pearse, 1980; Stallibrass, 1989). One difficulty with an individually based enhancement program is that it is most likely not cost efficient. An alternative is to deal with a larger social or ecological group (Allen, 1991; Castillo-Salgado, 1984; Stokols, 1992).

Education

One alternative to an individual client based mode of program delivery is to adopt an education approach (Cowen, 1991; Tones, 1986; WHO Regional Office for Europe, 1986a). As Cowen (1991) has suggested the obvious place to intervene is in the public school system, by establishing programs to teach children skills and attitudes that will enhance their competence. Another possibility, is to design curricula, so that, personality dispositions conducive to future enhancements to quality of life, can be modeled in the schools. For those beyond the school age, it is still possible to provide educational programs in the work place, or through continuing education classes. Calvert and Cocking (1992) have provided an interesting discussion of the use of media in the modification of lifestyles, and the enhancement of quality of life. There is a growing literature on the use of the media in health promotion, but space does not permit a review of this literature here. To date the results are not as impressive as might be expected, given the common expectation that the media are influential in shaping our sexual and aggressive behaviour. Perhaps, with more potent, well produced media interventions, greater effects will be acquired.

Legislation

A set of ecological groupings that has an impact on all our lives is government, local, state, federal, and international. Government action to implement programs that might enhance quality of life can be top-down, or bottom-up. In the top-down situation the particular government may think a program is a good idea (vote getter), and pass legislation or develop government policy to implement it. An example of such a top-down policy document is Epp's (1986) *Achieving Health For All: A framework for health promotion*. In the bottom-up situation social action may be required by the constituents to persuade government to enact legislation to implement a program (Tones, 1987). As Kickbusch (1987) and Tones (1986) have indicated the bottom-up approach may require consciousness raising, lobbying and advocacy. The WHO Regional Office for Europe (1986b) has provided an extensive list of the policy strategies, that can be used by governments, and the sectors in which programs can be developed with the goal of enhancing quality of life. As Castillo-Salgado (1984) has pointed out, there are four general tools a government can use to provoke changes that will result in enhanced quality of life. They are Education, Subsidization (reward activities that will enhance quality of life), Taxation (activities that will decrease quality of life), and Regulation (seat belt legislation). Stokols (1992) has provided an extensive discussion of the actual and potential actions of governments at various levels to involve themselves in programs to enhance quality of life.

The mechanics of introducing interventions to enhance quality of life are perhaps better understood than the specific intervention components that are required. There is ample evidence, that if a given program, with a particular orientation and mode of program delivery is identified as important, the expertise and technology for its implementation already exists in areas such as medicine, psychology, education, and government. As the previous sections of the chapter have underscored, there is a need to carry out extensive empirical research, that is both longitudinal, and based in the population at large. What must be evaluated are models such as the one depicted in Figure 1 so that the components that must go into programs to enhance quality of life can be determined. As

Stokols (1992) has argued, this research is required before substantial resources are committed to programs to enhance quality of life.

Recommendations:

1. Establish education programs at all levels (Kindergarten through Continuing Education) to help individuals develop healthy dispositions.
2. Establish education programs at all levels to help individuals develop general and domain specific life skills.
3. Establish support groups for individuals at risk for diminished quality of life.
4. Establish programs to modify the biosociophysical environment to enhance quality of life.
5. Reorient the current health (illness) system to provide HEALTH assessments, and interventions to enhance quality of life.
6. Develop media programs to model and foster healthy dispositions and life skills.

NOTES

Numerous students at The University of Western Ontario at the B.A., M.A., and Ph.D. level, who have assisted me with the research base for this chapter over the years are thanked for their contributions.

I wish to thank Sir David Williams, and the Fellows of Wolfson College for their collegial support during my sabbatical during which the initial literature review for this chapter was completed.

My thanks to Drs. A. C. Lindsay, D. R. Boughner, and F. N. McKenzie for making it possible for me to write this chapter, and to Dr. M. T. Hearn for enhancing my quality of life.

REFERENCES

Abbey, A. and F. M. Andrews: 1986, 'Modelling the psychological determinants of life quality', in F. M. Andrews (ed.), Research on the Quality of Life (The University of Michigan, Ann Arbor, MI).

Ackerman, N. M., G. O. Jenson and D. V. Bailey: 1991, 'Domains explaining the life quality of dairy farm couples', Lifestyles 12, pp. 107–130.

Allan, J. D. and B. A. Hall: 1988, 'Challenging the focus on technology: A critique of the medical model in a changing health care system', Advances in Nursing Science 10, pp. 22–34.

Allen, L. R.: 1991, 'Benefits of leisure services to community satisfaction', in B. L. Driver, P. J. Brown, and G. L. Peterson (eds.), Benefits of Leisure (Venture, State College, PA).

Andrews, F. M.: 1991, 'Stability and Change in levels and structure of subjective well-being: USA 1972 and 1988', Social Indicators Research 25, pp. 1–30.

Andrews, F. M., A. Abbey and L. J. Halman: 1991, 'Stress from infertility, marriage factors, and subjective well-being of wives and husbands', Journal of Health and Social Behaviour 32, pp. 238–253.

Bech, P.: 1990, 'Measurement of psychological distress and well-being', Psychotherapy and Psychosomatics 54, pp. 77–89.

Benum, K. and T. Anstorp: 1987, 'Social network stimulation. Health promotion in a high risk group of middle-aged women', Acta Psychiatrica Scananavica 76 (Suppl. 337), pp. 33–41.

Berry, R. E. and F. L. Williams: 1987, 'Assessing the relationship between quality of life and marital and income satisfaction: A path analytic approach', Journal of Marriage and the Family 49, pp. 107–116.

Bigelow, D. A., M. J. Gareau and D. J. Young: 1990, 'A quality of life interview', Psychosocial Rehabilitation Journal 14, pp. 94–98.

Brandtstädter, J. and B. Baltes-Götz: 1990, 'Personal control over development and quality of life perspectives in adulthood', in P. B. Baltes, and M. M. Baltes (eds.), Successful Aging: Perspectives from the Behavioral Sciences (Cambridge University Press, Cambridge).

Brief, A. P. and J. M. Atieh: 1987, 'Studying job stress: are we making mountains out of molehills?', Journal of Occupational Behaviour 8, pp. 115–126.

Brief, A. P., A. H. Butcher, J. M. George and K. E. Link: 1993, 'Integrating bottom-up and top-down theories of subjective well-being: The case of health', Journal of Personality and social Psychology 64, pp. 646–653.

Brown, R: 'Aging, disability and quality of life: A challenge for society', Canadian Psychology 30, pp. 551–559.

Campbell, A., P. E. Converse and W. L. Rodgers: 1976, The Quality of American Life: Perceptions, Evaluations, and Satisfactions (Russell Sage, New York).

Castillo-Salgado, C.: 1984, 'Assessing recent developments and opportunities in the promotion of health in the American workplace', Social Science and Medicine 19, pp. 349–358.

Chaturvedi, S. K.: 1991, 'What's important for quality of life to Indians – in relation to cancer', Social Science and Medicine 33, pp. 91–94.

Cheng, S. T.: 1988, 'Subjective quality of life in the planning and evaluation of program', Evaluation and Program Planning 11, pp. 123–134.

Chibnall, J. T. and R. C. Tait: 1990, 'The quality of life scale: A preliminary study with chronic pain patients', Psychology and Health 4, pp. 283–292.

Chubon, R. A.: 1987, 'Development of a quality-of-life rating scale for use in health-care evaluation', Evaluation and the Health Professions 10, pp. 186–200.

Cocking, R. R.: 1992, 'Implications of environmental variables for the quality of life', Journal of Applied Development Psychology 13, pp. 119–120.

Costa, P. T. and R. R. McCrea: 1980, 'Influence of extraversion and neuroticism on subjective well-being: Happy and unhappy people', Journal of Personality and Social Psychology 38, pp. 668-678.

Costa, P. T., R. R. McCrea and A. B. Zonderman: 1987, 'Environmental and dispositional influences on well-being: Longitudinal follow-up of an American national sample', British Journal of Psychology 78, pp. 299–306.

Cowen, E. L.: 1991, 'In pursuit of wellness', American Psychologist 46, pp. 404–408.

Csikszentmihalyi, M.: 1990, Flow: The Psychology of Optimal Experience (Harper and Row, New York).

Csikszentmihalyi, M. and J. LeFevre: 1989, 'Optimal experience in work and leisure', Journal of Personality and Social Psychology 56, pp. 815–822.

Davis, E. E. and M. Fine-Davis: 1991, 'Social indicators of living conditions in Ireland with European comparisons', Social Indicators Research 25, pp. iii–365.

De Groot, A. D.: 1986, 'An analysis of the concept of "Quality of Life"', in V. Ventafridda, F. S. A. M. van Dam, R. Yancik, and M. Tamburini (eds.), Assessment of Quality of Life and Cancer Treatment (Elsevier, Amsterdam).

Diener, E.: 1984, 'Subjective well-being', Psychological Bulletin 95, pp. 542–575.

Diener, E., R. A. Emmons, R. J. Larsen and S. Griffin: 1985, 'The Satisfaction With Life Scale', Journal of Personality Assessment 49, pp. 71–75.

Epp, J.: 1986, Achieving health for all: A framework for health promotion (Minister of Supplies and Services Canada, Ottawa).

Evans, D. R.: 1993, 'The Quality of Life Questionnaire in Practice, Program Evaluation, and Health Promotion', Paper presented at the annual meeting of the Ontario Psychological Association, Toronto, February 11–13.

Evans, D. R., G. Austin and M. Gemeinhardt: 1981, Microtraining and the enhancement of the Quality of Working Life (Research Bulletin No. 534) (The University of Western Ontario, Department of Psychology, London, Canada).

Evans, D. R., J. E. Burns, W. E. Robinson and O. J. Garrett: 1985, 'The Quality of Life Questionnaire: A multidimensional measure', American Journal of Community Psychology 13, pp. 305–322.

Evans, D. R. and W. E. Cope: 1989, Quality of Life Questionnaire Manual (Multi-Health Systems, Toronto).

Evans, D. R., M. T. Hearn, L. M. L. Levy and L. A. Shatford: 1989, 'Modern health technologies and quality of life measures', in R. C. King, and J. K. Collins (eds.), Social Applications and Issues in Psychology (Elsevier, North Holland).

Evans, D. R., M. T. Hearn, M. R. Uhlemann and A. E. Ivey: 1993a, Essential Interviewing; A Programmed Approach to Effective Communication 4th ed. (Brooks/Cole, Pacific Grove, CA).

Evans, D. R., A. B. Thompson, G. B. Browne, R. M. Barr and W. B. Barton: 1993b, 'Factors associated with the psychological well-being of adults with acute leukemia in remission', Journal of Clinical Psychology 49, pp. 153–160.

Evans, D. R., J. R. Pellizzari, B. J. Culbert and M. E. Metzen: 1993c, 'Personality, marital and occupational factors associated with quality of life', Journal of Clinical Psychology 49, pp. 477–485.

Faden, R. and A. Leplège: 1992, 'Assessing quality of life: Moral implications for clinical practice', Medical Care 30, pp. MS166–MS175.

Fava, G. A.: 1990, 'Methodological and conceptual issues in research on quality of life', Psychotherapy and Psychosomatics 54, pp. 70–76.

Frey, D. and C. J. Carlock: 1989, Enhancing Self Esteem 2nd ed. (Accelerated Development, Muncie, IN).

Frey, D. and C. J. Carlock: 1991, Practical Techniques for Enhancing Self-Esteem (Accelerated Development, Muncie, IN).

Frisch, M. B., J. Cornell, M. Villanueva and P. J. Retzlaff: 1992, 'Clinical validation of the Quality of Life Inventory: A measure of life satisfaction for use in treatment planning and outcome assessment', Psychological Assessment 4, pp. 92–101.

George, L. K.: 1992, 'Economic status and subjective well-being: A review of the literature and an agenda for future research', in N. E. Cutler, D. W. Gregg, and M. P. Lawton (eds.), Aging, Money, and Life Satisfaction (Springer, New York).

Goodinson, S. M. and J. Singleton: 1989, 'Quality of life: a critical review of current concepts, measures and their clinical implications', International Journal of Nursing Studies 26, pp. 327–341.

Grant, D., D. Evans, M. Hearn, J. Duff, C. Ghent and W. Wall: 1990, 'Quality of life after liver transplantation', Canadian Journal of Gastroenterology 4, pp. 49–52.

Groenland, E.: 1990, 'Structural elements of material well-being: An empirical test among people on social security', Social Indicators Research 22, pp. 367–384.

Gross, B. M.: 1966, 'Preface: A historical note on social indicators', in R. A. Bauer (ed.), Social Indicators (MIT Press, Cambridge MA).

Headey, B., R. Veenhoven and A. Wearing: 1991, 'Top-down versus bottom-up theories of subjective well-being', Social Indicators Research 24, pp. 81–100.

Headey, B. and a. Wearing: 1988, 'The sense of relative superiority - central to well-being', Social Indicators Research 20, pp. 497–516.

Headey, B., and A. Wearing: 1989, 'Personality, Life events, and subjective well-being: Toward a dynamic equilibrium model', Journal of Personality and Social Psychology 57, pp. 731–739.

Headey, B., and A. Wearing: 1990, 'Subjective well-being and coping with adversity', Social Indicators Research 22, pp. 327–349.

Headey, B., and A. Wearing: 1991, 'Subjective well-being: a stocks and flows framework', in F. Strack, M. Argyle, and N. Schwarz (eds.), Subjective Well-being: An Interdisciplinary Perspective (Pergamon, Oxford).

Hearn, M. T., L. A. Shatford, A. A. Yuzpe, S. E. Brown and R. F. Casper: 1987a, 'Psychological correlates of successful outcome in an in vitro fertilization program', Paper presented at the annual meeting of the American Psychological Associated, New York, August.

Hearn, M. T., A. A. Yuzpe, S. E. Brown and R. F. Casper: 1987b, 'Psychological characteristics of in vitro fertilization participants', American Journal of Obstetrics and Gynaecology 156, pp. 269–274.

Hoopes, L. L. and L. L. Lounsbury: 1989, 'An investigation of life satisfaction following a vacation: A domain-specific approach', Journal of Community Psychology 17, pp. 129–140.

Hughey, J. B. and J. W. Bardo: 1987, 'Social psychological dimensions of community satisfaction and quality of life: Some obtained relations', Psychological Reports 61, pp. 239–246.

Jenkins, C. D.: 1992, 'Assessment of outcomes of health intervention', Social Science and Medicine 35, pp. 367–375.

Johnston, D. F.: 1988, 'Toward a comprehensive 'Quality-of-Life' Index', Social Indicators Research 20, pp. 473–496.

Kaplan, R. M.: 1991, 'Assessment of quality of life for setting priorities in health policy', in H. E. Schroeder (ed.), New Directions in Health Psychology Assessment (Hemisphere, New York).

Karlsson, G.: 1992, 'The health economist's point of view concerning quality of life', Nordic Journal of Psychiatry 46, pp. 95–99.

Keller, R. T.: 1987, 'Cross-cultural influences on work and nonwork contributors to quality of life', Group and Organization Studies 12, pp. 304–318.

Kickbusch, I.: 1987, 'Issues in health promotion', Health Promotion 1, pp. 437–442.

King, K. B., L. A. Porter, L. H. Norsen and H. T. Reis: 1992, 'Patient perceptions of quality of life after coronary artery surgery: Was it worth it?', Research in Nursing and Health 15, pp. 327–334.

Kozleski E. B. and D. J. Sands: 1992, 'The yardstick of social validity: Evaluating quality of life as perceived by adults without disability', Education and Training in Mental Retardation 27, pp. 119–131.

Lance, C. E., G. L. Lautenschlager E. E. Sloan and P. E. Varca: 1989, 'A comparison between bottom-up, top-down, and bidirectional models of relationships between global and life facet satisfaction', Journal of Personality 57, pp. 601–624.

Latten, J. J.: 1989, 'Life-course and satisfaction, equal for every-one?', Social Indicators Research 21, pp. 599–610.

Lazarus R. S.: 1991a, 'Cognition and Motivation in emotion', American Psychologist 46, pp. 352–367.

Lazarus, R. S.: 1991b, Emotion and Adaptation (Oxford University Press, New York).

Lazarus, R. S.: 1993, 'Coping Theory and Research: Past, Present and Future', Psychosomatic Medicine 55, pp. 234–247.

Lazarus, R. S. and S. Folkman: 1984, Stress Appraisal, and Coping (Springer, New York).

Leslie, L. A. and E. A. Anderson: 1988, 'Men's and Women's participation in domestic roles: Impact on quality of life and marital adjustment', Journal of Family Psychology 2, pp. 212–226.

Loscocco, K. A. and A. R. Roschelle: 1991, 'Influences on the quality of work and In nonwork life: Two decades in review', Journal of Vocational Behaviour 39, pp. 182–225.

Matarazzo, J. D.: 1992, 'Psychological testing and assessment in the 21st century', American Psychologist 47, pp. 1007–1018.

McCulloch, D.: 1991, 'Can we measure 'output'? Quality-adjusted life years, health indices and occupational therapy', British Journal of Occupational Therapy 54, pp. 219–221.

McGee, H. M., C. A. O'Boyle, A. Hickey, K. O'Malley and C. R. B. Joyce: 1991, 'Assessing the quality of life of the individual: The SEIQoL with a healthy and a gastroenterology unit population', Psychological Medicine 21, pp. 749–759.

Mugenda, O. M., T. K. Hira and A. M. Fanslow: 1990, 'Assessing the causal relationship among communication, money management practices, satisfaction with financial status, and satisfaction with quality of life', Lifestyles 11, pp. 343–360.

O'Brien, B. J., N. R. Banner, S. Gibson and M. H. Yacoub: 1988, 'The Nottingham Health Profile as a measure of quality of life following combined heart and lung transplantation', Journal of Epidemiology and Community Health 42, pp. 232–234.

Ouellette-Kuntz, H.: 1990, 'A pilot study in the use of the Quality of Life Interview Schedule', Social Indicators Research 23, pp. 283–298.

Palys, T. S. and B. R. Little: 1980, 'Social indicators and the quality of life', Canadian Psychology 21, pp. 67–74.

Parasuraman, S., J. H. Greenhaus, S. Rabinowitz, A. G. Bedeian and K. W. Mossholder: 1989, 'Work and family variable as mediators of the relationship between wives' employment and husband's well-being', Academy of Management Journal 32, pp. 185–201.

Pavot, W. and E. Diener: 1993, 'Review of the Satisfaction With Life Scale', Psychological Assessment 5, pp. 164–172.

Pearse, I. H.: 1980, 'The Quality of Life: The Peckham Approach to Human Ethology 2nd ed. (Scotish Academic Press, Edinburgh).

Pellizzari, J. R.: 1992, 'An integration of several conceptions of well-being: Subjective well-being, quality of life, motivational and positive psychological functioning approaches', Unpublished master's thesis, The University of Western Ontario, London, Ontario, Canada.

Pellizzari, J. R. and D. R. Evans: 1991, 'Personal growth and quality of life', Paper presented at the annual meeting of the Canadian Psychological Association, Calgary, Alberta, June.

Pellizzari, J. R. and d. R. Evans: 1992, 'Personal strivings, subjective well-being, and quality of life', Paper presented at the annual meeting of the Canadian Psychological Association, Quebec City, Quebec, June.

Poloma, M. M. and B. F. Pendleton: 1990, 'Religious domains and general well-being', Social Indicators Research 22, pp. 255–276.

Rettig, K. D., S. M. Danes and J. W. Bauer: 1991, 'Family life quality: Theory and assessment in economically stressed farm families', Social Indicators Research 24, pp. 269–299.

Rice, R. W.: 1984, 'Organizational work and the overall quality of life', Applied Social Psychology Annual 5, pp. 155–178.

Rice, R. W., M. R. Frone and D. B. McFarlin: 1992, 'Work-nonwork conflict and the perceived quality of life', Journal of Organizational Behaviour 13, pp. 155–168.

Romney, D. M., C. D. Jenkins and J. M. Bynner: 1992, 'A structural analysis of health-related quality of life dimensions', Human Relations 45, pp. 165–176.

Russell, R. V.: 1990, 'Recreation and quality of life in old age: A causal analysis', Journal of Applied Gerontology 9, pp. 77–90.

Ryff, C. D.: 1989, 'Beyond Ponce de Leon and Life satisfaction: New directions in the quest for successful ageing', International Journal of Behavioral Development 12, pp. 35–55.

Scheier, M. F., K. A. Matthews, J. F. Owens, G. J. Magovern, R. C. Lefebvre, R. A. Abbott and C. S. Carver: 1989, 'Dispositional optimism and recovery from coronary artery bypass surgery: The beneficial effects on physical and psychological well-being', Journal of Personality and Social Psychology 57, pp. 1024–1040.

Sheets, V. L. and C. D. Manzer: 1991, 'Affect, cognition, and urban vegetation: Some effects of adding trees along city streets', Environment and Behaviour 23, pp. 285–304.

Spilker, B., F. R. Molinek, K. A. Johnston, R. L. Simpson and H. H. Tilson: 1990, 'Quality of life bibliography and indexes', Medical Care 28, pp. DS1–DS77.

Stallibrass, A.: 1989, Being Me and Also Us: Lessons from the Peckham Experiment (Scotish Academic Press, Edinburgh).

Stokols, D.: 1992, 'Establishing and maintaining health environments: Toward a social ecology of health promotion', American Psychologist 47, pp. 6–22.

Sullivan, L. W.: 1991, 'Partners in prevention: A mobilization plan for implementing Health People 2000', American Journal of Health Promotion 5, pp. 291–297.

Sullivan, M.: 1992, 'Quality of life assessment in medicine: Concepts, definitions, purposes, and basic tools', Nordic Journal of Psychiatry 46, pp. 79–83.

Thomas, M. E. and M. Hughes: 1986, 'The continuing significance of race: A study of race, class, and quality of life in America, 1972–1985', American Sociological Review 51, pp. 830–841.

Tolman, E. C.: 1941, 'Psychological Man', Journal of Social Psychology 13, pp. 205–218.

Tones, B. K.: 1986, 'Health education and the ideology of health promotion: a review of alternative approaches', Health Education Research 1, pp. 3–12.

Waltz, M. and B. Badura: 1988, 'Subjective health, intimacy, and perceived self-efficacy after heart attack: Predicting life quality five years afterwards', Social Indicators Research 20, pp. 303–332.

Watson, D., L. A. Clark and A. Tellegen: 1988, 'Development and validation of brief measures of positive and negative affect: The PANAS scales', Journal of Personality and Social Psychology 54, pp. 1063–1070.

WHO Regional Office for Europe: 1986a, 'A discussion document on the concept and principles of health promotion', Health Promotion 1, pp. 73–76.

WHO Regional Office for Europe: 1986b, 'A framework for health promotion policy: A discussion document', Health Promotion 1, pp. 335–340.

Williams, R. L., M. Eyring, P. Gaynor and J. D. Long: 1991, 'Development of Views of Life Scale', Psychology and Health 5, pp. 165–181.

Woodruff, S. I. and T. L. Conway: 1992a, 'A longitudinal assessment of the impact of health/fitness status and health behaviour on perceived life quality', Perceptual and Motor Skills 75, pp. 3–14.

Woodruff, S. I. and T. L. Conway: 1992b, 'Impact of health and fitness – related behaviour on quality of life', Social Indicators Research 25, pp. 391–405.

World Health Organization: 1947, Constitution of the World Health Organization (Geneva, Author).

Young, M. Y.: 1991, 'The adjustment of Salvadorian refugees: Stressors, resources and well-being', Unpublished doctoral dissertation, The University of Western Ontario, London, Ontario, Canada.

University of Western Ontario,
Department of Psychology,
London, Ontario,
Canada

MARCIA G. ORY AND DONNA M. COX

FORGING AHEAD: LINKING HEALTH AND BEHAVIOR TO IMPROVE QUALITY OF LIFE IN OLDER PEOPLE

(Accepted 14 February, 1994)

ABSTRACT. This chapter will focus on conceptual and methodological issues related to health promotion/disability prevention for older people. The first section will begin with a discussion of why older people, as compared to younger persons, are not traditionally seen as targets of health promotion efforts. In recent years several national working groups have been established to examine how older people's health and functioning can be improved. Their objectives and recommendations for older Americans will be reviewed. The second section will address the conceptual framework underlying health and behavior research supported by the National Institute on Aging. The movement from correlational studies to studies of basic mechanisms linking health and behaviour will be discussed, with particular attention to interactions with aging processes. Examples of health and behavior research representing these processes will be presented as well as methodological issues in the measurement of health and functional outcomes for older people. Measurement of quality of life in the cognitively impaired is seen as especially difficult. The third section will review several common themes emanating from these research studies. These include attention to a life course perspective, variability in aging processes, alternative research approaches, and intervention strategies for both initiating and maintaining recommended behavioral changes. A fourth section will review current areas of investigation at the National Institute of Aging. Successful intervention strategies in both community and institutional settings will to presented. These include: (1) a comprehensive behavioral and environmental falls prevention program which has been shown to reduce falls in the community; (2) a health education program to increase older women's use of cancer-related health practices; and (3) behavioral strategies for reducing incontinence in nursing homes. A new NIA initiative on special care units for persons with dementia will also be discussed. The fifth and final section will deal with issues involved in the translation of research into policy and practice. Approaches for increasing the relevance of research to policymakers will be discussed.

Social Indicators Research **33**: 89–120, 1994.
© 1994 *Kluwer Academic Publishers. Printed in the Netherlands.*

HEALTH CARE AND THE HEALTH CARE NEEDS OF OLDER PEOPLE

Demographic trends, coupled with ideological and economic concerns, are revolutionizing the American health care system. The 1990s have brought increased attention to aging, health care and quality of life issues. The current debate on health care reform in the United States is fueled by concerns that the existing system is not adequate to provide health care for the burgeoning numbers of Americans who need care. Despite the huge sums of dollars spent on health care in the United States, older people's fundamental concerns about health, health care and quality of life remain largely unaddressed. The aging of the population can be viewed as a demographic time bomb that will only increase health care demand and costs.

Developed and developing nations throughout the world are experiencing an unprecedented increase in the number of people who live to the age of 65 and beyond. In 1992, approximately 342 million people (6.2%) across the globe were aged 65 and over. This number represented an absolute increase of 9.7 million people since 1991 (U.S. Bureau of the Census, 1992). Though Europe has the highest proportion of elderly people (14% in 1990), North American populations are not far behind. By the year 2008, 14% of Canada's population will be 65 years and older, and the U.S. is expected to reach that mark by 2012. Between 1990 and 2025, the percent increase in the Canadian and U.S. elderly population is expected to be 141% and 101%, respectively (U.S. Census, 1992). Though they constitute a very small portion of the world population, people who are 85 years and older are of special concern particularly in the U.S. Currently, this "oldest-old" group (85+) represents nearly 10% of all elderly in the U.S. and is expected to triple in size between now and 2030 (U.S. Census, 1992; U.S. Census, 1993).

The dramatic increases in life expectancy are largely due to declines in mortality among the middle-aged and elderly populations. In 1900, a 65-year old person could expect to live nearly 12 more years; today, the 65-year old could expect to live more than 17 years (U.S. Bureau of the Census, 1993). Yet, decreases in mortality are not without consequences. Most older people are not frail and dependent as aging stereotypes depict; with increased longevity however, increases in the number of chronic diseases are followed by increases in death and disability due to chronic disease (Institute of Medicine, 1991). Just in the last decade, the number of multiple chronic conditions reported by older people have notably increased. With most older people now reporting two or more chronic conditions, older women are especially likely to experience multiple chronic conditions, in contrast to older men (Rice, 1989; Guralnik et al., 1989). The increases in chronic conditions often translate into functional disability and need for some type of assistance (Verbrugge, 1990). Approximately 7 million Americans over the age of 65 depend on others for help with some basic task of daily living (Ory and Duncker, 1992).

Projections of life expectancy now differentiate years of active life expectancy or healthy years of life from the number of expected years of life. For example, a healthy male who reaches age 65 can expect to live at least 15 more years, but good health and independence may be expected for only 13 of those extra years (Suzman et al., 1992). A healthy woman, on the other hand, can expect to live as many as 20 more years after reaching age 65 but may enjoy good health for just 16 of those years. Since the ill health of older persons is not necessarily a fixed intrinsic process related to biological senescence, but rather the result of the cumulative exposure to risk (Suzman et al., 1992), research on aging includes the identification of ways to *enhance* the quality of one's life rather than to simply extend it.

As years of life expectancy increase, a review of issues and problems associated with quality of life in these final years becomes crucial. Quality of life is a concept that often alludes to evaluations of some component of life specifically, or life overall. It is a concept with special significance in light of medical and technological advances which have important implications for how disease and treatment affect the lives of people (Stewart and King, 1991).

Since older people can expect to live well into their 80s, there is sufficient time for interventions directed at health promotion to have an effect on improving quality of life and functional status (Omenn, 1992). Therefore, the crux of the issue is how research can be directed toward understanding health behaviors for the purpose of developing interventions that keep older people healthy and independent for as long as possible.

OVERVIEW OF CHAPTER

Section one of this chapter will begin with a focused discussion of conceptual and methodological issues related to health promotion/disability prevention for older people and the implications for quality of life research. These introductory remarks will include a discussion of why older people, as compared to younger populations, are not traditionally seen as targets of health promotion efforts. Also included in this portion of the chapter will be a review of the objectives and recommendations of several national working groups, established to examine how the health and functioning of older Americans can be improved. Sections two through five will include: (1) a discussion of the conceptual framework underlying health and behavior research supported by the National Institute on Aging; (2) a review of common themes emanating from these research studies; (3) a review of four current areas of investigation at the National Institute on Aging, and (4) a discussion of issues involved in translating research into policy and practice to improve quality of life.

SECTION I: INCORPORATING THE AGING DYNAMIC IN THE CONCEPTUALIZATION AND MEASUREMENT OF QUALITY OF LIFE

Living longer has important implications for quality of life, particularly for the individual whose extra years of life are marked by illness, declining health, social isolation and reduced independence. Longer lives filled with increased illness and disability will place added burdens on social and medical services, thus escalating health care costs.

Aging and Quality of Life

However, recent findings from a longitudinal analysis of older people's health and functional status between 1982 and 1989 (Manton *et al.*, 1993a) suggest that population aging does not inevitably lead to increases in disability rates. Manton and colleagues provide strong support for the "compression of morbidity" hypothesis (e.g. as people age, fewer years of disability will be experienced by older people because illness and associated disability will be postponed until the latest stages of life).

Despite an increase in the number of aged individuals, significant declines were found in the number of individuals who had difficulty performing specific daily activities, such as eating, bathing, dressing, as well as instrumental activities such as cooking, shopping and managing finances (Manton et al., 1993b). Changes were also noted in services used by disabled people (e.g., increases in certain equipment) suggesting the importance of social and physical environment in determining whether particular functional impairments and disabilities are translated into handicaps.

This research has important implications for research to maintain and even improve the quality of an aging individual's life. There is a dynamic interplay of social, behavioral and biomedical processes which accumulate over a lifetime to impact the health and functioning of older persons. Specific groups distinguished by demographic and social factors, such as race, gender and socio-economic factors, may not experience the same level of functional change, if any. Racial and ethnic diversities that are compounded by dissimilar life-long patterns of health and health care generate diverse health experiences. This observed variability in the aging process along with changing social conditions demonstrates that the process of aging is malleable and subject to some degree of human intervention and control (Riley and Riley, 1989).

Measuring quality of life, therefore, becomes extremely important for acquiring baseline information for comparisons of different groups over time, and especially for evaluating the effectiveness of programs/interventions aimed at improving quality of life. The concept of quality of life is multidimensional and includes factors related to the domains of physical health, social functioning, emotional well-being and general health perceptions. Each domain is affected by the events and situations of an older person's life and each will have a bearing on an assessment of quality of life. It is extremely important to keep domains separate because the evaluation of one can be very different from another. For example, though an older person may assess social functioning positively, an objective assessment of physical functioning may be less than expected (Ory, 1988).

However, variability within older groups and between younger age groups create special challenges for measuring an older person's quality of life. Older populations are distinctive from younger age groups by virtue of their life experiences and values. Age-related factors affecting older people's health and social situations further complicate the measurement of quality of life in this group.

First, the subjective component of quality of life measurement requires that an older person be able to express feelings, perceptions, etc. If an older person becomes cognitively impaired, other ways must be found to tap this very important aspect of measurement.

Second, quality of life measurement instruments used for younger populations are not necessarily appropriate for use with older people. For example, some instruments which measure depression (e.g., Center for Epidemiologic Studies-Depression Scale [CES-D]) combine physical and psychological components. As already pointed out, assessments of physical functioning and psychological well-being may be very different for the older person.

Finally, the sensitivity of the quality of life measurement becomes an issue if scales do not adequately capture the extremes. For example, since older people can expect to have more than one chronic disease that together produce variable levels of disability, measurement scales must be sensitive to the diversity which exists within disabled groups of older people. These scales must be able to identify and distinguish between older people who are considered to be "very healthy" (e.g., few to no chronic disease with associated disability) versus those who are designated as "very disabled" (e.g., multiple chronic diseases and associated disabilities) (Kutner *et al.*, 1992).

Aging and Health Promotion

As noted previously, the dynamic nature of the aging process suggests that it can be changed to reduce negative outcomes and favor positive ones (Riley *et al.*, 1987). Therefore, health promotion efforts to maintain function are extremely important as one ages because most old people do experience at least one chronic condition. Hence, putting aside popular assumptions and stereotypes about older people and the aging process are important precursors to enhancing older people's quality of life.

Health promotion is not usually thought to be associated with ideas about aging. In contrast to health promotion efforts that are directed at younger people, interventions to promote health in the aged have traditionally been considered as occurring too late to be effective. There has been a supposition that behavioral or lifestyle changes in late life have only a minimal impact on health and functioning. Stereotypes cast older people as inflexible, unwilling or unable to change health attitudes, behaviors or lifestyles. In addition, health promotion interventions (i.e., drug or exercise regimens) have historically been thought to be too strenuous for older people to tolerate (Ory, 1988; IOM, 1990).

Recent research shows the fallaciousness of these ageist assumptions (Ory et al., 1992). The changes in attitudes toward older people and health promotion can be seen in three national health promotion efforts undertaken in the United States in the late 1980s and early 1990s. In 1988, The Office of the Surgeon General called together a first national workshop on health promotion and aging. This workshop resulted in a set of health promotion research, education and service recommendations related to alcohol, oral health, physical fitness and exercise, injury prevention, medications, nutrition, preventive health services, and smoking cessation (Office of the Surgeon General, 1988).

Two other federal activities in the early 1990s called further attention to the importance of health promotion for older people. After conducting a decade review of national health promotion and disease prevention goals, the Department of Health and Human Services (DHHS, 1990) revised its Year 2000 goals for older people to include more health promotion and prevention objectives. The Institute of Medicine (IOM) (1990) also commissioned a special committee to examine what was known about promoting health and preventing disability in the last fifty years of life. These efforts have resulted in expanding the definition of health promotion in older people to include prevention efforts across the entire health and illness continuum (e.g., primary, secondary and tertiary prevention).

The central purpose of each of these efforts has been to examine how the health and functioning of Americans can be improved. Each has been important for establishing priorities, recommending areas for further research and identifying educational and service programs needed to improve the health and functioning of older people today. The most important aspect of these U.S. health promotion efforts is the recognition that older people can be educated to detect and seek treatment of health conditions (e.g., heart disease and cancer); that older people can and should play an active part in the health professional's care and treatment plan (i.e., joint involvement in clinical decision-making); and that behavior and attitudes can be changed to positively affect health.

SECTION II: HEALTH AND BEHAVIOR RESEARCH

Research identifying how social and behavioral factors interact with biological factors to influence health and functioning in the middle and later years makes a significant contribution to the emergent field of psychosocial geriatric research (Ory *et al.*, 1992). Such research adds to our understanding of how the conceptualization and thus, measurement of quality of life changes as people age and face different life situations.

In 1979, the U.S. Surgeon General's Report *Healthy People* (U.S. Department of Health Education and Welfare, 1979) directed the national spotlight on the relationship between health and behavior by documenting the extent to which lifestyles contributed to the burden of chronic illness in the United States and other industrialized countries. The importance of health behaviors and lifestyle factors is clearly noted in the *Healthy People 2000* (DHHS, 1990) objectives for the nation. The significance of this area of research is evident in its increased visibility within research priorities at the National Institutes of Health. For examples, health and behavior research is now an integral part of the National Institute of Aging's congressional mandate for understanding the aging process and the dynamics of change.

Pathways Linking Health and Behavior

Traditionally, most studies have identified the epidemiological associations between health and behavior. Research attention is now needed to specify the direct and indirect linkages between health and behavior. Three types of bio-behavioral processes have been identified to link behavior to physical or mental illness (Abeles, 1988, p. 3–4):

(1) health-impaired habits and lifestyles such as smoking, heavy drinking, lace of exercise, poor diet, and poor hygienic practices;

(2) reactions to illness, including delays in seeking medical care, minimizing the significance of symptoms, and failing to comply with treatment and rehabilitation regimens; and

(3) direct alterations in tissue function through the brain's influence on hormone production and other physiological responses to psychosocial stimuli, particularly stress.

Social and behavioral factors are associated with a wide range of outcomes and are believed to play a role in the onset and course of disease. It may be that social factors affect general susceptibility to disease or that they affect survival. For example, the presence of social support may be seen as an important factor in survival and recovery such as stroke, hip fractures (Vogt et al., 1992). The wide range of outcomes associated with social and behavioral conditions suggests that a number of pathways lead from social and behavioral factors to illness and/or that certain factors act to increase general susceptibility to disease (Berkman, 1989; Cassel, 1976).

There are several schema to help understand the relations between health and behavior. While some are more complicated in their representation, each examines direct and indirect social and behavioral processes, intervening physiological pathways and various stages in the onset and course of disease processes and outcomes.

Conceptual Models

A simplified schema (Fig. 1) to illustrate linkages between health and behavior suggests a single pathway from health-related behaviors (attitudes and behaviors) to health outcomes through intervening physiological or psychosocial variables (i.e., reactions to illness). This simplified schema is useful, but does not capture the dynamic interaction between health and behavior. Therefore, an expanded schema (Fig. 1b) incorporates several facets not specifically identified in the earlier schematic illustration:

- the influence of exogenous social and environmental factors on health related behaviors and intervening variables;
- the separation of health attitudes from health behaviors, psychosocial from physiological mediators and biological effects from health/disease outcomes;
- attention to interactions between physical and mental health; and
- recognition of reciprocal relationship (e.g., one's state of health can influence health-related behaviors or intervening processes).

A third representation (Fig. 2) is more complex but it includes the role of aging and hypothesizes several possible pathways through which age influences the relationship between health and behavior. This schema more clearly elucidates the dynamic nature of the aging process, heavily influenced by different aspects of aging (i.e., biological, cognitive, attitudinal, motivational and social).

The various pathways point to the influence of particular behaviors and attitudes on the health of people as they age; the ways in which health attitudes and behaviors interact with physiological and psychological aging processes, and the impact of the socio-cultural environment on the development, maintenance and potential modification of attitudes and behaviors. For example, since people are shaped by the structure of groups and surrounding social systems, norms and expectations related to health behavior and expectations will differ for groups of older people depending on the time period and/or social conditions in which they

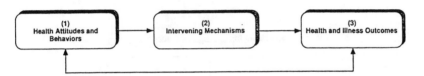

Fig. 1. Health and behavior linkages: (A) A simplified schema.

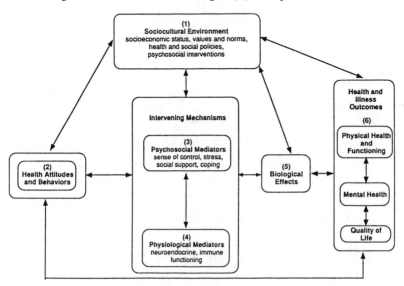

Fig. 1 (B) An expanded schema.

live. The socio-cultural environment, often ignored in most health and behavior models, imposes powerful age-based regulatory norms and social-structural arrangements that follow an entirely different set of attitudes. These socio-cultural processes and changes, still largely neglected in aging research, are the focus of a current NIA-supported PROJECT AGE AND STRUCTURAL CHANGE ("PASC").[1]

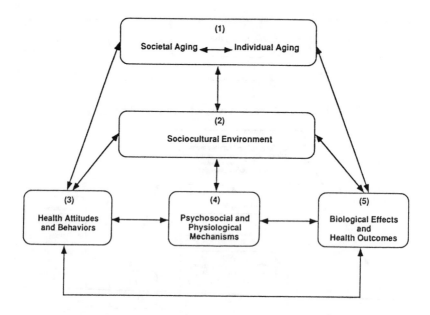

Fig. 2.   Schema of aging, health, and behavior linkages.

Research Areas and Illustrative Findings

Four categories for research on health and behavior have been developed by the NIH Working Group on Health and Behavior (Abeles, 1990)
to illustrate how the aging process is affected by the aging, health and
behavior linkages represented in Fig. 3.

Identification and distribution of psychosocial risk factors. This category for research on health and behavior includes research on correlations between (a) particular behavioral, social, and cultural factors and
(b) various aspects of health and functioning. In addition, the spectrum and prevalence of such factors in different population groups are
considered. The basic question for this research is whether risk factors
identified in middle age populations hold for older populations.

For example, in a follow-up study of adults 40 years and older who
participated in a 1965 mail survey of physical, social and psychological

indicators of health conducted by the Human Population Laboratory of the California Department of Health Services in Alameda county, California, health behaviors and social conditions have been found to change over the life course with predictable impacts noted on subsequent mortality risks (Kaplan and Haan, 1989). Follow-up investigations have found the same basic risk factors in old age as in younger populations. Smoking, physical inactivity, poor eating habits and social isolation are each related to mortality risks. Social and behavioral factors are also powerful predictors of functional outcomes throughout the life course (Kaplan and Strawbridge, 1994, in press). The findings empirically challenge the idea that an 80 year old man will not benefit from smoking cessation or increases in physical activity. Therefore, one can never assume that it is too late to stop health impairing habits (e.g., smoking) or to start new healthy ones (e.g., exercise).

This type of longitudinal study also provides an opportunity to look at the natural history of risk factors. We can see how health behaviors cluster together, how they change over time and what these changes may suggest about morbidity and mortality rates. In the Alameda study, for instance, many changes in basic risk factors which have been noted are a reflection of increased public awareness of and secular changes in attitudes toward preventive health and healthy living. Changes toward more healthy practices are associated with more positive outcomes and vice versa. The clustering of specific negative health behaviors also suggests groups who are least likely to adopt healthy practices (e.g., smokers and sedentary adults).

Research in the area of behavioral epidemiology suggests that the meaning of some risk factors may change with aging, or be different as a consequence of differences in the aging experiences of groups. Consider social support for example. In general, the presence of social support has been considered an important factor for better health, particularly for older people. This association has been demonstrated through research. More recent research is specifying the influence of different types of social support on both the onset and course of illness. In a study of Health Maintenance Organization (HMO) enrolles, 18 years and older, who were followed for 15 years, Vogt and colleagues (1992) examined different constructs of social support in terms of size, scope and frequency to determine their relation to morbidity and mortality. Research results suggest that social support has a powerful association with survival in the presence of chronic disease, particularly for older people.

Even within the older population, interesting relationships have been found to suggest that the health of some groups relies more on specific types of social support (e.g., the presence of a spouse) than others. This is true in the case of men and women. Since women live longer than men, they are most likely to be widowed in old age. Yet, the associations between marital status and mortality that are present for older men are not present for older women (Kaplan and Haan, 1989). Women are likely to identify and rely on different sources of social support as they age. In addition, specific roles of women, such as kinkeepers, or the multiple roles assumed in a lifetime may broaden the network of available supports for women, making it more likely and/or easier for relationships with others to be effectively substituted when spouses are no longer available (Moen *et al.*, 1992).

Development, maintenance, and change of health-related behaviors. This category focuses on research of particular health-related behaviors, such as smoking or sedentary lifestyle, and the antecedent factors establishing, maintaining, and altering these behaviors. The goal is to understand the mechanisms by which behaviors correlated with negative health and functioning outcomes can be prevented or changed, and how behaviors correlated with positive outcomes can be supported.

There are a number of interesting studies in this area that are contributing to a range of information that is especially important for improving quality of life of older people. One particular study has focused on self-care behaviors. At the Cecil G. Sheps Center for Health Services Research at the University of North Carolina, DeFriese and colleagues will provide needed information on the extent and ways in which self-care activities of older adults maintain independent living status despite the presence of significant functional limitations. The design of the study permits the first-ever examination of a nationally-representative sample of both well and frail elderly persons of all age groups in rural and urban areas (DeFriese, 1992).

The majority of health-related behaviors are in fact self-care behaviors. Self-care behaviors are defined to include a broad range of activities that a person uses to maintain and promote health, and to prevent, detect, and treat health problems. This includes health practices (i.e., smoking, eating, exercise), knowledge and use of preventive items (e.g., first aid kits, smoke alarms, etc.) and responses to both acute and chronic conditions (that is, how people adapt and manage functional limitations).

The National Self-Care Study revealed that a significant proportion of the older population engage in one of three types of self-care behaviors (e.g., alter daily routines and behaviors, use special equipment or receive help from others to perform daily activities (DeFriese and Woomert, 1992). Importantly, the practice of health promotion and disease prevention behaviors seems to be widespread in the population of community-based older: 56% get adequate sleep; 88% eat breakfast regularly; 77% avoid eating between meals; 58% maintain appropriate body weight; 96% either never drink or have moderate alcohol consumption (no more than two drinks in a sitting); 55% have never smoked cigarettes; and 68% remain physically active with sports, walks, gardening or other forms of exercise (DeFriese, 1992).

Other studies focus on identifying factors which will improve older people's quality of life. For example, no existing epidemiologic study of aging, in women or men, provides the range of direct physiological, social and behavioral data that a new study being conducted in a semi-rural city north of San Francisco will produce. Using a full census of all persons 55 years and older, Tager and colleagues (1992) at the University of California, San Francisco will provide the largest data set on the physical functioning of men and women, and associated physiological factors that relate to level of function and potential for increased function. The study will examine if lowered levels of exercise capacity and pulmonary function are important predictors of sex-specific, age-related lowered levels of, and more rapid declines in self-reported and objectively measured physical performance. It will also examine the role of social and cognitive factors in modifying actual sex-specific physical performance in relationship to physiological potential. Moreover, unlike existing studies, this study will provide data on several hundred women between the age of 55–64 years, an important age group for understanding changes that take place in women in later decades. The data from this study will fill a void by providing data on physical fitness in older women and on the capacity of older women to improve their fitness.

Stereotypes of aging have an important influence on health attitudes and behaviors. Though we know that frailty and decline is not an inevitable aspect of aging, there is still much work to be done to successfully distinguish between images and perceptions of what is believed to be "normal" aging and symptoms that are associated with illness. Perceptions of what is "normal" interfere with early detection and treatment of disease. Older people tend to ignore symptoms (i.e., pain, fatigue), or if reported are likely to have reported symptoms ignored by health professionals who attribute them to "growing old" (Kart, 1981; Prohaska et al., 1987). This inattention to symptoms more than likely delays treatment which can have a host of negative consequences. For example, many older women experience problems with urinary incontinence. Yet they are unlikely to seek help for what is often a treatable condition because they have come to believe that it is a normal part of aging. What is even worse is that those who do bring their complaints to the attention of their physicians or other health professionals are often told that nothing can be done (Mitteness, 1990). The appropriate recognition and treatment of chronic conditions, often thought to be a consequence of "normal aging", is one of NIA's primary goals.

An interesting line of research in this area but one which is fraught with confusion, is how older people cope with illness and stress in their lives. There are two schools of thought on this subject. The first suggests that older people cope less effectively than other age groups because they are worn down by the cumulative stresses and strains during their life. An alternative view contends that older people in fact cope more effectively because they have learned useful coping strategies over the course of a lifetime. Others have suggested that differences between the two schools of thought may be accounted for by whether or not the coping strategy used is effective for a particular situation and a particular point in time. To date, research seems to indicate that coping with illness depends more on the specific illness or disability the older persons faces than on the patient's age per se (Kiyak and Borson, 1992).

Basic biobehavioral mechanisms. This is an area of research which stresses the mechanisms or processes through which behavior influences, and is influenced by, health and illness. The emphasis is on identifying the physiological processes that explain the correlations identified by psychosocial risk-factor analyses (e.g., the effects of stress on health through changes in immune functioning). Currently, this is a particularly important area for research because information is limited. Promising research is beginning to develop, however. Particularly interesting research in this area are studies of how stress associated with factors such as caregiving or older people's sense of control, influence health and immune functioning.

For example, research on the identification of caregiver burden and stress has mounted in recent years. However, there is now a new focus which attempts to understand what effects caregiving stress has on immune functioning (Kiecolt-Glaser, in press). This emphasis moves research beyond the identification and description of general burdens to *how* burdens contribute to changes in immune functioning and specific parameters of health.

A second example of social and behavioral research on immune functioning suggests a general model of how an individual's sense of control is related to health (Rodin and Timko, 1992). The model looks at intervening physiological processes and asks what difference age makes. Rodin and colleagues at Yale suggest that sense of control over one's environment affects health outcomes in two major ways: (1) by affecting health related behaviors and (2) by direct physiological effects on neuroendocrine and immune responses. Research suggests that there are detrimental effects on the health and quality of life of older people when their control over activities is restricted and that interventions which enhance options for control promote health. However, it is of importance to note that individual preferences for control differ widely and variability for preferred levels of control may increase with age (Lachman and Ziff, 1994, in press; Baltes, 1994, in press).

Behavioral and social interventions to prevent and treat illness or to promote health. This is an area of research which uses findings from research areas previously discussed to develop and evaluate behavioral and social interventions (e.g., clinical trials, field experiments). Research shows that many health conditions associated with aging, such as urinary incontinence or falls, can be prevented or ameliorated (Schnelle, 1992; Hornbrook *et al.*, 1993). Although long-term maintenance effects remain illusive, the effectiveness of various behavioral and social interventions is being demonstrated through randomized experimental designs with standardized protocols and outcome measurements. This area is of particular importance when discussing quality of life because research is applied for the purpose of improving health outcomes and evaluated to determine how effective a strategy is in achieving the goals.

SECTION III: COMMON THEMES IN AGING RESEARCH

There are several important themes present in this area of research. First, social and behavioral interventions incorporate the life course perspective as a fundamental building block. An objective is to change risk factors with aging but there is recognition of the effects of risks accumulated over a lifetime. It is important to consider the influence of early childhood practices and current activities on outcomes, as well as to identify windows of vulnerability over the lifecourse. Though changes in health behavior occur in later life, they do not necessarily translate into better health. There may be critical periods of exposure to risk which influence health and functioning outcomes. For example, poor eating habits in young life may have an influence on weight and health in later life even though diet practices have improved over time (Ory, 1988; Ory *et al.*, 1992).

Second, though the individual is commonly thought to be the focus of interventions, the community and/or society as a whole may be the target of such research. Many health conditions are the product of person-environment interactions. The socio-cultural environment must be included in research as an important variable when examining people's behavior and health (Riley and Riley, 1989; Levi and Cox, 1994). Moreover, health behaviors are very complex. In developing interventions to prevent disease/promote health, objectives may require the elimination of several undesirable practices; learning and encouragement of new practices that will promote health and; the incorporation and maintenance of those practices as part of a new lifestyle for the individual (Rakowski, 1992). Processes associated with the initial adoption of a behavior may be very different from those influencing the long-term incorporation of a behavior into one's lifestyle. For example, people may initiate exercise programs to improve physical fitness but they will only continue if exercise programs are convenient.

Finally, research in this area must adhere strongly to principles about variability and heterogeneity of aging. An intervention developed for young-old white, urban populations may be problematic if applied to rural, non-white groups and most likely will not produce the same results. Therefore, there has been an extensive effort in recent years by NIH, and particularly NIA, to refocus research attention on the individual characteristics and needs of specific groups in the population, such as women, minorities, ethnic populations and the oldest old.

SECTION IV: CURRENT AREAS OF RESEARCH

Encouraging Physical Activity and Reducing Frailty

Reducing frailty and injury prevention is an area of special interest and importance to those concerned with quality of life issues. More than 25% of older people in the community fall every year. Fall-related injuries are associated with enormous costs. Maintaining, or even improving the strength, mobility, balance and endurance of older people to preserve their capabilities in performing normal daily activities and reducing risks of falls and other associated traumas, is an important priority of research supported by the NIA.

Regular physical activity is now recognized as a critical element in the prevention of disease and enhancement of health in adulthood (King *et al.*, 1993). Knowledge that behaviors can change makes it possible to apply what is known about behaviors and attitudes for the purpose of developing interventions to facilitate behavioral and attitudinal changes to improve health outcomes. There are some excellent examples of this type of applied research in the area of physical fitness/activity. Behavioral interventions have been developed that increase exercise and physical activity with positive results (Buchner *et al.*, 1993; Stevens *et al.*, 1992; Hornbrook *et al.*, 1993). However, there is still much to learn about the role of regular exercise in preventing frailty and institutionalization in old age.

In a Stanford University study, Haskell and colleagues (1992) are currently examining how well physical activity regimens targeted to community living elders can achieve changes in physical performance and other health-related indices across an extended time period. This project provides an unique opportunity for evaluating physical activity measures in older people and assessing the quality of life effects of physical activity training regimens. The research project is especially important for its careful attention to theoretical and practical issues in achieving program adherence which will assist other researchers to design and implement community-wide health intervention studies in older populations. Other research which is focused on identifying the best strategies for improving activity (e.g., exercise regimens performed in the home versus those performed in groups, or high-intensity programs versus low-intensity programs) suggest that health problems and preferences for various formats in exercise are strong factors in determining continued participation in community-based programs (King *et al.*, 1993).

Other important research in this area includes the Multicenter Trials of Frailty and Injuries: Cooperative Studies of Intervention Techniques (FICSIT), a project supported under a cooperative agreement for 1990–1993 by the National Institute on Aging and the National Institute of Nursing Research. FICSIT is a series of randomized clinical trials of biomedical, behavioral, and environmental interventions designed to increase physical functional capacity and reduce falls and fall-related injuries among the elderly. Sample sizes range from 100 to 1250. Each clinical center collects its own site-specific data, while simultaneously contributing to a large body of data common to all sites (Ory *et al.*, 1993; Hadley *et al.*, 1993).

The trials involve an innovative mix of exercise, nursing, prevention, and rehabilitation techniques. Exercise programs represent a continuum, ranging from the ancient Oriental practice of Tai Chi to high-intensity aerobic dance programs. Rehabilitation strategies, including physical conditioning and educational programs, are aimed at creating an awareness of behavioral risks and environmental hazards.

The multi-center trials established quality of life as an important mediator of compliance and intervention effectiveness, as well as an important outcome variable. Interventions to increase physical functioning capacity may have differential effects on various domains of quality of life (e.g., emotional or social function). These effects may increase or decrease a person's compliance with a regimen (i.e., increasing activity may increase a person's fear of falling and injury; participation in a exercise program may increase a person's perception of social support and decrease depressive symptoms). Therefore, the incorporation of quality of life measures in the multi-center trials provided important data to examine compliance and predict treatment success (Kutner et al., 1992).

Increasing Preventive Health Behaviors in Older Women

Older women are at higher risk of breast cancer but are less likely to be screened (Costanze, 1992; Rimer et al., 1992). A series of studies were conducted in different communities, using different interventions. Some interventions (e.g., education, mass media, mobile vans) focused on changing behaviors in older women; others focused on physicians. In one community, mobile vans (to reduce transportation barriers) and intensive educational efforts were used to increase mammogram use (Rimer, 1991). Since the study was conducted before the implementation of the 1991 Medicare Mammogram benefit, the investigators provided subsidized mammograms to simulate the anticipated Medicare situation.

In collecting data about older women's cancer-related beliefs and behaviors, researchers found that older women were not generally aware of their increased risk for breast cancer. Prior to implementation of the intervention, the oldest women were the least likely to have discussed mammogram with their physicians or to indicate an intention to obtain one in the next year. A majority of older women also held the erroneous belief that a mammogram was unnecessary if one felt fine. Such beliefs were significantly associated with mammography usage.

The intervention (Rimer, 1991) was highly successful in increasing older women's use of mammogram. Compared to 12% of women in the control group who were just given a subsidy, 45% of the women who were provided a subsidy and participated in a tailored health program for older women had a mammogram during the intervention period. Controlling for confounding health beliefs, further analyses indicated that women due for a mammogram at the intervention sites were six times more likely to obtain one than women who had not participated in the educational program.

Despite the significant intervention effect, a majority of older women still did not avail themselves of the opportunity to receive a mammogram. The under-utilization of breast cancer screening has significant implications for women's quality of life in the later years. First of all, metastatic breast cancer is a disabling and very painful disease (Cassel, 1992). Secondly studies have shown that age at time of diagnosis seems to have an effect on recuperation time (Satariano, 1990). Older women experience longer recuperating periods for physical problems than younger women and are least likely to be independent in instrumental activities of daily living (IADL), such as housekeeping, meal preparation, shopping for groceries. Therefore, early diagnosis of breast cancer not only delays death but it also impacts the quality of a woman's additional years of life after diagnosis.

Improving Quality of Life in Nursing Homes: Maintaining Continence

A series of collaborative clinical trials co-sponsored by NIA and the National Institute of Nursing Research demonstrate the potential for behavioral treatment for managing urinary incontinence in older persons (NIH, 1988). A simple nursing management protocol based on behavioral principles such as prompted voiding, social reinforcement and toileting assistance has been shown to reduce significantly urinary incontinence, even in severely impaired nursing home patients. In this series of studies, researchers are: (a) identifying which groups of older people are most responsive to treatment; (b) examining the cost-effectiveness of such interventions, and (c) identifying organizational factors that affect staff compliance (Hu *et al.*, 1989; Schnelle *et al.*, 1989).

For example, the trials suggest the need for defining what is meant by "success." Is the intervention only a success if subjects remain dry or does success constitute some measure of improvement in incontinence? Whose perspective is most important in defining "success" ... the perspective of the health professional or that of the older woman? These are important questions when evaluating an intervention. Individuals differ in their preferences. A woman with a major incontinence problem may be happy with reduced number of episodes. On the other hand, those with rare occurrences but active lifestyles, may want more assurance.

It has come as a surprise that urinary incontinence can be kept to a minimum in nursing homes. If residents are asked if they need toileting assistance every two hours, about 70% show improvement and 30–35% of residents can be kept mostly dry (Schnelle *et al.*, 1991). Research has shown that a lot of urinary incontinence in a nursing home is a function of the care provided, rather than a health condition specific to the resident. If residents could get to a toilet, they would not become incontinent. Though nursing home standards suggest that residents are checked and changed every two hours, this is not the case. Random checks in nursing homes show that residents are often wet for extended periods of time.

However, the development of an intervention that can decrease resident incontinence does not necessarily imply that the nursing home's incontinence problem has been resolved. The central focus of intervention applied in institutional settings must be on staff adherence. The health care environment must be examined and a system found that will motivate staff to use the regimens. An effective implementation of the regimens also requires that very specific performance standards be set. A study (Schnelle *et al.*, 1993) which focused on redesigning the way in which nursing assistants and nurses worked together found that dryness could be maintained in residents for up to six months, at least among the most responsive residents. Schnelle and associates devised a management program of prompted voiding care routines based on quality control technology that is used in business and industry. Nurse managers were provided with an easy way of checking compliance, thereby making nursing assistants' performance more visible. This series of studies has demonstrated empirically that long-term maintenance can be achieved by reinforcing successful behavioral strategies with new systems of staff training and management based on statistical quality control techniques.

Enhancing Care for Persons with Dementia: Special Care Units

A final example illustrating current emphases in social and behavioral research focuses on specialized institutional care for persons with Alzheimer's disease. Both researchers and practitioners concerned with issues related to the quality of care in nursing homes have suggested that residents with dementia might benefit from specially designed programs or environments. Such distinct sections or programs within nursing homes are commonly known as "special care units". Special care units (SCUs) have proliferated across the U.S. in recent years, but very little is known about the relative advantages and disadvantages associated with this type of care setting, or how these programs compare to traditional nursing home care in terms of costs and effectiveness.

In response to the need for information about SCUs, the National Institute on Aging established the Special Care Unit (SCU) Initiative in 1991 to undertake a systematic study of the characteristics and effects of SCUs on residents with Alzheimer's disease (AD) or related dementias. Modest research efforts in the past point out crucial research questions and methodologies needed to appropriately evaluate SCUs. The SCU Initiative is the first multi-site national study to examine the positive and negative consequences of SCUs on residents and others involved in their care. Under this initiative, NIA has funded ten research projects to study SCUs throughout the United States. While each of the ten studies has unique features, investigators from each study collaborate on such issues as, defining what constitutes an SCU, determining how residents with dementia will be identified, and evaluating how care in SCUs affects the residents, nursing home staff and family caregivers.

The ten studies will examine systematically different aspects of care as they may affect residents with dementia, their family members and health care administrators and practitioners.

The ultimate goal of the NIA SCU Initiative is to determine the extent to which "special care" improves the quality of life of an individual with Alzheimer's disease or related dementias, as well as that of the individual's family. The SCU Initiative will (1) determine if and how SCUs improve the quality of care provided to residents with dementia and their families, and (2) provide public policymakers with the necessary information to assist the decision-making process, particularly in respect to regulatory and reimbursement issues. The Initiative is part of a wider research effort within NIH which examines the social and health care needs of people with AD. It pulls together two of NIA's top priorities – Alzheimer's disease and long term care and will be important in the identification of the best and most cost-effective way to care for people with Alzheimer's disease or related dementias.

SECTION V: TRANSLATION OF RESEARCH INTO POLICY/PRACTICE FOR IMPROVING QUALITY OF LIFE

Thus far, this paper has focused on the conceptualization and measurement of quality of life with particular attention given on health and behavior research for enhancing life throughout the life course. Despite the promise of current and future health promotion and rehabilitation research, any success towards improving quality of life for groups of older people will be limited if the information is not effectively communicated or deemed to be relevant by practitioners, program administrators or policy makers. Often research results that have program or policy implications are ignored by these vested interests. But, there are ways to increase the relevance of research to policy makers.

First, when identifying important problems for study, researchers should consider the significance of findings for the individual *and society*. The macro-level perspective will promote some awareness of the ramifications of expected findings on broader issues as they relate to different groups and/or society in general. At some later date, this exercise will facilitate the translation of research as relevant to practitioners and policy makers. In addition, intervention research should build from what is known and demonstrate some potential for application with many groups, or the potential for modification with similar success across groups.

Second, practical solutions that can be incorporated into existing systems must be developed by researchers. This is especially important for research within institutional settings. An intervention can only be successful if it is correctly implemented and produces expected results over the long term. If the required personnel and other resources are beyond the scope of the institution, the intervention will have no practical use to the organization, its personnel or its clients.

Third, some balance must exist between clinical experience and population-based research if research is to have any practical policy application. While it is important to appreciate clinical impressions and experience, clinicians often see a very select part of the population. The every day experiences of the population are very different from what occurs in a clinical setting.

Fourth, interventions should be developed from theoretical frameworks that identify underlying mechanisms and social conditions necessary for the intervention to be successful. Knowledge that an intervention can improve quality of life is not sufficient. The practical application of research requires an understanding of *why* it works. This knowledge makes it possible to identify specific situations when an intervention will be effective and suggests which aspects require modification for the same success if applied to other settings. Most importantly, information regarding the practical applications of research must be communicated to policymakers. Therefore, researchers must be sensitive to language. Using scientific jargon with peers is expected; using it with policymakers will confuse and complicate, as well as increase the likelihood that useful information will be ignored.

Finally, researchers must be concerned about the timeliness of studies and results. Using ongoing studies to "piggyback" new research questions to examine other timely issues are important.

The goal of good research should be not only to increase knowledge bases but to apply knowledge for the benefit of individuals in society.

This goal is evident in social and behavioral research on aging which promotes health for the purpose of improving the quality of life of the aging individual, whether that person lives in the community or in a nursing home. Research studies, such as those discussed in this chapter, have effectively demonstrated the malleability of the aging process, as well as the variability of aging experiences. This knowledge has been instrumental in laying aside many of the stereotypical images and ideas associated with aging. However, there is still much to do.

Bridges between clinical settings and the practical world must continue to be strengthened. Further development of the lines of communication between the research community and policymakers is recommended. If the needs of modern society are to be met, it is imperative that the research community and policymakers become partners with a similar goal ... the betterment of life for all members of society.

NOTES

[1] Under the leadership of Matilda White Riley, PASC focuses on understanding *structural* opportunities and constraints that affect the quality of aging from birth to death. It is an area of research which needs further conceptual, methodological and substantive understanding. The effort will bring into the social science approach both demography and biology and lead to a dynamic and multi-disciplinary bio-psychosocial model with an emphasis on mechanisms through which relations among different subsystems are maintained.

REFERENCES

Abeles, R. P.: 1988, 'Health and Behavior Research Initiatives by the National Institutes of Health, FY 1989', Unpublished report prepared for the Department of Health and Human Services and submitted to the Senate committee on Appropriations for the Departments of Labor, Health and Human Services, and Education, and Related Agencies.

Abeles, R. P.: 1990, 'Health and Behavior Research Initiatives by the National Institutes of Health', Unpublished report prepared for the Department of Health and Human Services and submitted to the Senate Committee on Appropriations for the Departments of Labor, Health and Human Services, and Education, and Related Agencies.

Aging America: Trends and Projections: 1991, Prepared by the U.S. Senate Special Committee on Aging, the American Association of Retired Persons, the Federal Council on the Aging and the U.S. Administration on Aging. Washington, D.C.

Baltes, M. M.: 1994, in press, 'Aging well and institutional living: a paradox?', in R. P. Abeles, H. C. Gift and M. G. Ory (eds. with the assistance of D. M. Cox), Aging and Quality of Life: Charting New Territories in Behavioral Sciences Research (Springer Publishers, New York).

Berkman, L.: 1989, 'Maintenance of Health, prevention of disease, a psychosocial perspective', in National Center for Health Statistics, Health of an Aging America: Issues on Data for Policy Analysis, Vital and Health Statistics, Series 4, No. 25, DHHS Pub. No. [PHS] 89–1488 (Government Printing Office, Washington, D.C.), pp. 39–55.

Buchner, D. M., M. C. Hornbrook, N. G. Kutner, M. E. Tinetti and M. G. Ory: 1993, 'Development of the common data base for the FICSIT trials', Journal of the American Geriatrics Society 41(3), pp. 297–308.

Cassel, J.: 1976, 'The contributions of the social environment to host resistance', American Journal of Epidemiology 104(2), pp. 1072–1123.

Cassel, C. K.: 1992, 'Breast cancer screening in older women: ethical issues', presented at the Forum on Breast Cancer Screening in Older Women, Sturbridge, MA. August 1, 1990. Journals of Gerontology 47 (Special Issue), pp. 121–125.

Costanza, M. E. (Ed.): 1992, 'Breast Cancer Screening In Older Women', Journals of Gerontology 47 (Special Issue).

DeFriese, G. H.: 1992, 'Self-care assessment of the community-based elderly persons project' (Cooperative Agreement AG07929–03), Unpublished report to the National Institute on Aging.

DeFriese, G. H. and A. Woomert.: 1992, 'Informal and formal health care systems serving older persons', in M. G. Ory, R. P. Abeles and P. D. Lipman (eds.), Aging, Health and Behavior (Sage Publications, California).

Guralnik, J. A., A. Z. LaCroix, D. F. Everett and M. G. Kovar: 1989, 'Aging in the Eighties: The prevalence of comorbidity and its association with disability', National Center for Health Statistics, May 26, 170.

Haskell, W. L.: 'Community Exercise Training in Older Women and Men', Unpublished report, National Institute on Aging Grant R01 AG09991.

Hornbrook, M. C., V. J. Stevens, D. J. Wingfield, J. F. Hollis, M. N. Greenbeck and M. G. Ory: 1993, 'Preventing falls among community dwelling older persons: results from a randomized trial', The Gerontologist 3, pp. 16–23.

Hu, Teh-Wei, J. F. Igou, L. Kaltreider, L. D. Yu, T. J. Rohner, P. J. Dennis, W. E. Craighead, E. C. Hadley and M. G. Ory: 1989, 'A clinical trial of a behavioral therapy to reduce urinary incontinence in nursing homes: outcomes and implications', The Journal of the American Medical Association 261, pp. 2656–2662.

Institute of Medicine: 1990, The Second Fifty Years: Promoting Health and Preventing Disability (National Academy Press, Washington, D.C).

Institute of Medicine: 1991, 'Extending life, enhancing life', A National Research Agenda on Aging (National Academy Press, Washington, D.C).

Kaplan, G. A. and W. J. Strawbridge: 1994 (in press), 'Behavioral and social factors in healthy aging', in R. P. Abeles, H. C. Gift and M. G. Ory (eds. with the assistance of D. M. Cox), Aging and Quality of Life: Charting New Territories in Behavioral Sciences Research (Springer Publishers, New York).

Kaplan, G. A. and M. N. Haan: 1989, 'Is there a role for prevention among the elderly? epidemiological evidence from the alameda county study', in M. G. Ory and K. Bond (eds.), Aging and Health Care (Routledge, New York).

Kart, C.: 1981, 'Experiencing Symptoms: Attribution and Misattribution of Illness Among the Aged', in M. R. Haug (ed.), Elderly Patients and Their Doctors (Springer-Verlag, New York).

Kiecolt-Glaser, J. K. and R. Glaser: in press, 'Caregivers, Mental Health and Immune function', in E. Light and B. Lebowitz (eds.), Advances in Alzheimer's Disease Caregiving and Family Stress (Springer, New York).

King, A. C., W. L. Haskell, C. Barr Taylor, H. C. Kraemer and R. F. DeBusk: 1991, 'Group- vs Home-Based Exercise Training in Healthy Older Men and Women', Journal of the American Medical Association 266(11), pp. 1535–1542.

King, A. C., C. Barr Taylor and W. L. Haskell: 1993, 'Effects of Differing Intensities and Formats of 12 Months of Exercise Training on Psychological OUtcomes in Older Adults', Health Psychology Journal 12(4), pp. 292–300.

Kiyak, A. H. and S. Borson: 1992, 'Coping with Chronic Illness and Disability', in M. G. Ory, R. P. Abeles and P. D. Lipman (eds.), Aging, Health and Behavior (Sage Publications, California).

Kutner, N. G., M. G. Ory, D. I. Baker, K. B. Schechtman, M. C. Hornbrook and C. D. Mulrow: 1992, 'Quality of life assessment issues in a health-promotion intervention trial with older people', in Public Health Reports 107(5), pp. 530–539.

Lachman, M. E., M. A. Ziff and A. Spiro III: 1994 (in press), 'Maintaining a sense of control in later life', in R. P. Abeles, H. C. Gift and M. G. Ory (eds. with the assistance of D. M. Cox), Aging and Quality of Life: Charting New Territories in Behavioral Sciences Research (Springer Publishers, New York).

Levi, L. and D. M. Cox: 1994 (in press), 'Changing the social environment to promote health', in R. P. Abeles, H. C. Gift and M. G. Ory (eds. with the assistance of D. M. Cox), Aging and Quality of Life: Charting New Territories in Behavioral Sciences Research (Springer Publishers, New York).

Manton, K. G., L. S. Corder and E. Stallard: 1993a, 'Estimates of change in chronic disability and institutional incidence and prevalence rates in the U.S. elderly population from the 1982, 1984, and 1989 National Long Term Care Survey', Journal of Gerontology 48(4), pp. S153–S166.

Manton, K. G., L. S. Corder and E. Stallard: 1993b, 'Changes in the use of personal assistance and special equipment 1982–1989: Results from the 1982 and 1989 National Long Term Care Survey', The Gerontologist 33(2), pp. 168–176.

Mitteness, L. S.: 1990, 'Knowledge and beliefs about urinary incontinence in adult-hood', Journal of the American Geriatrics Society 38, pp. 374–378.

Moen, P., D. Dempster-McClain and R. M. Williams, Jr.: 1992, 'Successful aging: A life-course perspective on women's multiple roles and health', American Journal of Sociology 97(6), pp. 1612–38.

National Institutes on health: 1988, 'Urinary incontinence in adults', Consensus Development Conference Statement (Author, Bethesda, MD).

Office of the Surgeon General: 1988, Surgeon General's Workshop: Health Promotion and Aging: Proceedings of a Workshop (Government Printing Office, Washington, D.C.).

Omenn, G. S. (ed): 1992, 'Health promotion and disease prevention', Clinic in Geriatric Medicine.

Ory, M. G.: 1988, 'Considerations in the development of age-sensitive indicators for assessing health promotion', Health Promotion: An International Journal 3(2), pp. 139–150.

Ory M. G., R. P. Abeles and P. D. Lipman: 1992, 'Introduction: an overview research of aging, health and behavior', in M. G. Ory, R. P. Abeles and P. D. Lipman (eds.), Aging, Health and Behavior (Sage Publications, California).

Ory, M. G. and A. P. duncker: 1992, 'Introduction: the home care challenge', in M. G. Ory and A. P. Duncker (eds.), In-Home Care for Older People: Health and Supportive Services (Sage Publications, Newbury Park).

Ory, M. G., K. B. Schechtman, J. P. Miller, E. C. Hadley: 1993, 'Frailty and injuries in later life: the FICSIT trials', Journal of the American Geriatrics Society 48 (Special Issue) 41(3), pp. 283–296.

Prohaska, T. R., M. L. Keller, E. A. Leventhal and H. Leventhal: 1987, 'Impact of symptoms and aging attribution on emotions and coping', Health Psychology 6, pp. 495–514.

Rakowski, W.: 1992, 'Disease prevention and health promotion with older adults', in M. G. Ory, R. P. Abeles and P. D. Lipman (eds.), Aging, Health and Behyavior (Sage Publications, California).

Rice, D.: 1989, 'Demographics and health of the elderly: past trends and projections', Report to the Prospective Payment Advisory Committee.

Riley, M. W., J. D. Matarazzo and A. Baum (eds.): 1987, Perspectives in Behavioral Medicine: The Aging Dimension (Lawrence Erlbaum, Hillsdale, N. J.).

Riley, M. W. and J. W. Riley, Jr.: 1989, 'The quality of aging: strategies for interventions', The Annals of the American Academy of Political and Social Science 503, pp. 9–147.

Rimer, B. K., N. Tesch, E. King, C. Lerman, E. Ross, A. Boyce and P. F. Engstrom: 1992, 'The role of multi-strategy health education program in increasing mammography use among women 65+', Public health reports 107(4), pp. 369–380.

Rimer, B. K., E. Ross, C. Suzanne Cristinzio and E. King: 1992, 'Older women's participation in breast screening', Journals of Gerontology 47 (Special Issue), pp. 85–91.

Rodin, J. and C. Timko: 1992, 'Sense of control, aging and health', in M. G. Ory, R. P. Abeles and P. D. Lipman (eds.), Aging, Health and Behavior (Sage Publications, California).

Satariano, W. A., N. E. Ragheb, L. G. Branch, G. M. Swanson: 1990, 'Difficulties in physical functioning reported by middle-aged and elderly women with breast cancer: a case-control comparison', Journals of Gerontology 45, pp. M3–M11.

Schnelle, J. F., B. Traughber, V. A. Sowell, D. R. Newman, C. O. Petrelli and M. G. Ory: 1989, 'Prompted voiding treatment of urinary incontinence in nursing home patients: a behavioral management approach for nursing home staff', Journal of the American Geriatrics Society 37, pp. 1051–1057.

Schnelle, J. F., D. R. Newman, T. E. Fogarty, K. Wallston and M. G. Ory: 1991, 'Assessment and quality control of incontinence care in long-term nursing facilities', Journal of American Geriatrics Society 39, pp. 165–171.

Schnelle, J. F., D. R. Newman, M. White, J. Abbey, K. A. Wallston, T. E. Fogarty, M. G. Ory: 1993, 'Maintaining continence in nursing home residents through the application of industrial quality control', The Gerontologist 33(1), pp. 114–121.

Stevens, V. J., M. C. Hornbrook, D. J. Wingfield, J. F. Hollis, M. R. Greenlick and M. G. Ory: 1991/1992, 'Design and implementation of a falls prevention intervention for community- dwelling older persons', Behavior, Health and Aging 2(1), pp. 57–73.

Stewart, A. L. and A. C. King: 1991, 'Evaluating the efficacy of physical activity for influencing quality of life outcomes in older adults', Annals of Behavioral Medicine 13, pp. 108–116.

Suzman, R. M., D. P. Willis and K. G. Manton: 1992, The Oldest Old (Oxford University Press, New York).

Tager, I. B.: 1992, 'Epidemiology of aging and physical performance', National Institute on Aging Grant R01 AG09389.

U.S. Bureau: 1992, International Population Reports, P25, 92–3, An Aging World II (U.S. Government Printing Office, Washington, D.C.).

U.S. Bureau of the Census, Current Population Reports, Special Studies: 1993, P23–178, 'Sixty-five plus in America' (Government Printing Office, Washington, D.C.).

U.S. Department of health, Education and Welfare, Public Health Service: 1979, Healthy People: The Surgeon General's Report on Health Promotion and Disease Prevention (Government Printing Office, Washington, D.C.).

U.S. Department of Health, Education and Welfare, Public Health Service: 1980, Healthy People 2000: National Health Promotion and Disease Prevention Objectives for the Nation (Government Printing Office, Washington D.C.).

U.S. Department of Health and Human Services: 1990, Promoting Health/Preventing Disease: Year 2000 Objectives for the Nation (Government Printing Office, Washington, D.C.).

Verbrugge, L. M.: 1990, 'The iceberg of disability', in S. M. Stahl (ed), The Legacy of Longevity (Sage, Newbury Park, CA).

Vogt, T., J. Mullooly, D,. Ernst, C. Pope and J. Hollis: 1992, 'Social networks as predictors of ischemic health disease, cancer, stroke and hypertension: incidence, survival and mortality', Journal of Clinical Epidemiology 45(6), pp. 659–666.

Behavioral and Social Research,
National Institute on Aging,
Bethesda, MD 20892,
U.S.A.

ROBERT M. KAPLAN

USING QUALITY OF LIFE INFORMATION TO
SET PRIORITIES IN HEALTH POLICY

(Accepted 14 February, 1994)

ABSTRACT. Health care has as primary objectives extending life expectancy and improving quality of life in years prior to death. This paper offers a General Health Policy Model as a method for quantifying these outcomes. The model adjusts life expectancy for diminished quality of life, which is measured using a standardized instrument known as the Quality of Well-being (QWB) scale. The Well-year or Quality Adjusted Life Year (QALY) results from these analyses and serves as a single quantitative expression of health benefit. QALY units integrate side effects and benefits of treatment by combining into a single number, mortality, morbidity, and duration of each health state. Examples show the application of the model relevant to a variety of medical and public health problems, including diabetes, arthritis, AIDS, neonatal circumcision, and tobacco tax. It is suggested that the General Health Policy Model has advantages for guiding both individual and public health decisions.

Until recently, medical scientists did a poor job of documenting how their care affected people. Most of what medicine attempts to accomplish is not well represented by standard measures of morbidity and mortality. The traditional approach to reimbursement for health care services allowed physicians to select which procedures and tests they deemed were appropriate for their patients. Although decisions are supposed to be between a doctor and his/her patient, patients have been in a disadvantaged position. Because of their illness, patients may have limited information to challenge their physicians. Patients have also become less price conscious since the bills are often paid by a faceless insurance company. Yet increasing evidence suggests that the tests and procedures administered to many patients are not in their best interest (Brook and Lohr, 1986).

Social Indicators Research **33**: 121–163, 1994.
© 1994 *Kluwer Academic Publishers. Printed in the Netherlands.*

This chapter suggests that available resources be used to produce the greatest benefit for the greatest number of people. In the US, as much as 30 to 50% of expenditures in health care may have no effect upon health outcome (Brook and Lohr, 1986). Although there are no similar estimates for Canada, it is suspected that many non-efficacious procedures are in use. By denying coverage for these services and targeting those outcomes where treatment makes a difference, costs might be reduced or stabilized and the savings could be used to increase access. Most importantly, this is a new paradigm in which health outcomes are the pivotal dimension. The major challenge in executing this system is in defining what is meant by health benefit.

UTILITY

Utility is a condition or quality of usefulness. High utility items are the most useful and those with lower utility are less useful. States of being are also associated with utility and health is often identified as the highest utility asset. When Rokeach (1973) asked subjects to prioritize their values, he found no variability for the rank of health. It was always ranked first and, for this reason, was eventually removed from the Rokeach value scale. One of the purposes of this article is to define health and to offer a quantitative expression of health status.

Since good health is so highly valued, people will spend their energy and assets attempting to achieve it. In 1994, Americans spent an esti-mated 900 billion ($900 000 000 000) on health care services and a much larger amount on other products and services related to health. Although there is tremendous incentive to promote products and services as health enhancing, we typically are left with little information about the extent to which health outcome is affected by these investments. Thus, another purpose of this article is to evaluate improvements in health that may result from investments.

IS MORE BETTER?

One of the basic objectives in health care is to deliver service. Indeed, many policy options are justified because they provide more care. We assume that expenditure is an accomplishment. The more money allocated to a program, the better the expected outcomes. It is often assumed that the states or countries that are achieving the best health outcomes are those spending the most money. Thus, it might be argued, Americans should have the world's best health profile because they spend the most per capita on health care. However, that is not the case, at least according to common health indicators. Although Americans spend more on health care than any other country, they do not live longer than their economically equivalent counterparts and their infant mortality is higher, not lower (Kaplan, 1993).

Substantial evidence has emerged suggesting that many unnecessary services are delivered by our health care system. Consider coronary artery bypass surgery. The United States Congress Office of Technology Assessment reported that in France there are 19 such operations per million members of the population. In Austria, there are 150 operations per million in the population. In the United States, there are nearly 800 operations per million (Rimm, 1985). Approximately 200 000 procedures were performed in the United States in 1985 – nearly twice as many as had been performed in 1980 (National Center for Health Statistics, 1986). There are also large differences in the use of other expensive interventions. For example, the number of people with end-stage renal disease is believed to be approximately equal in western countries. Yet, in the United Kingdom, less than 1 case per 1 000 was on renal dialysis in comparison to 39 cases per 1 000 in the United States (Schroeder, 1987). As argued by a variety of analysts, there is no evidence that these regional variations in use of procedures has substantial effects on health outcomes. They do have systematic effects upon health care costs.

Policy analysts are faced with difficult choices because they hope to maximize health outcomes while maintaining control over costs. Western countries differ in the rate at which health care costs have escalated with the United States leading the pack in expenditures. It is not clear that escalating expenditure has been associated with equal returns in health status. Among European countries reporting data to the Organization for Economic Co-operation and Development the shortest life expectancies for men were in Ireland and the longest are in Greece. Among the reporting nations, Greece paradoxically spends the smallest percentage of their GNP on health care while Ireland spends the most. In fact, there is a rough negative relationship among the reporting nations between expenditures and life expectancy (Sick Health Services, 1988). Studies (reviewed by Voulgaropolous *et al.*, 1989) have shown that many widely used and expensive procedures have essentially no health benefit.

In order to gain a better understanding of the alternatives in health care, we have proposed a General Health Policy Model that attempts to provide a comprehensive expression of the costs, risks, and benefits of competing alternatives in health care. Some of these choices are difficult without a model because comparing programs might be considered analogous to comparing apples to oranges.

APPLES VERSUS ORANGES

There are many alternative ways to spend money on health care. These range from complex, high tech interventions such as liver transplantation, to rehabilitation, to primary prevention. Comparing these alternatives might be analogous to comparing apples to oranges. Further complicating the comparison is the fact that the benefits of each intervention are measured in quite different units. Liver transplantation might be evaluated in terms of extended life expectancy while a vaccination program might be evaluated by a reduction in school days missed. The successful liver transplantation procedure might be one in which the patient survives for one year. These procedures might require large expenditures for a single patient. The same amount of money might be spent to provide a different smaller benefit for a large number of people. Each liver transplant, for example, costs about $325 000 and it has been argued that public support for these procedures be abandoned in order to support programs such as prenatal care. Yet, the systematic comparison between the benefits of liver transplantation and prenatal care are not possible because the outcomes of the services were measured in quite different units. How can we compare apples to oranges? In the following sections, models for thinking about this problem will be discussed.

Public policy makers are faced with complex decisions that often involve comparisons between very different alternatives. When these alternatives are measured or described using different scales, decisions can be difficult, if not impossible. Often, the confused decision-maker gives in to the alternative with the most emotional appeal. In this chapter, it is argued that general measurement models, based on outcome measurement, can provide important new insights for policy makers. These models depend on very general conceptualizations of the expected benefits or consequences of health care decisions. The General Health Policy Model (Kaplan and Anderson, 1990, Kaplan, 1993, Kaplan *et al.*, 1993) that quantitatively expresses the ultimate objectives of health care–to extend life expectancy and to improve quality of life.

COMPARISONS ACROSS DIAGNOSES – THE INCREMENTAL OUTCOME PROBLEM

In order to resolve health care cost problems, we need formal decision-making models. Mathematical models of decision-making are now being proposed in a variety of health care systems. For example, these models have been suggested for use in European, New Zealand, Australian, and American health care systems. There is a growing recognition that health care resources are very limited. The United Kingdom National Health Service, for example, has recognized the need to prioritize competing demands on their very limited budgets (Maynard, 1991, Rosser, 1993). Yet prioritization schemes make little sense without some consideration of outcome.

The most important challenge in developing a formal model for resource allocation is in defining a common unit of health benefit. Typically, the value of each specific intervention in health care is determined by considering a measure specific to the intervention or the disease process. Treatments of hypertension, for example, are evaluated in terms of blood pressure while those for diabetes are evaluated by blood glucose. Yet it is difficult to compare the relative value of investing in blood glucose versus blood pressure reduction. Traditional public health measures, such as life expectancy, are usually too crude to allow appropriate prioritization. However, we believe a general model of health outcome is both feasible and practical.

A GENERAL HEALTH POLICY MODEL

In order to understand health outcomes, it is necessary to build a comprehensive theoretical model of health status. This model includes several components. The major aspects of the model include mortality (death) and morbidity (health-related quality of life). In several papers, we have suggested that diseases and disabilities are important for two reasons. First, illness may cause the life expectancy to be shortened. Second, illness may make life less desirable at times prior to death (health-related quality of life) (Kaplan and Anderson, 1990; Kaplan *et al.*, 1993).

Over the last two decades, a group of investigators at the University of California, San Diego, has developed a General Health Policy Model (GHPM). Central to the general health policy model is a general conceptualization of health status. The model separates aspects of health status into distinct components. These are life expectancy (mortality), functioning and symptoms (morbidity), preference for observed functional status (utility) and duration of stay in health states (prognosis).

A. *Mortality*

A model of health outcomes necessarily includes a component for mortality. Indeed, many public health statistics focus exclusively on mortality through estimations of crude mortality rates, age-adjusted mortality rates, and infant mortality rates. Death is an important outcome that must be included in any comprehensive conceptualization of health.

B. *Morbidity*

In addition to death, behavioral dysfunction is also an important outcome. The General Health Policy Model considers functioning in three areas: mobility, physical activity, and social activity. Descriptions of the measures of these aspects of function are given in many different publications (see Kaplan and Anderson, 1990, Kaplan, 1993). Most public health indicators are relatively insensitive to variations toward the well end of the continuum. Measures of infant mortality, to give an extreme example, ignore all individuals capable of reading this journal since they have lived beyond one year following their births (we assume that no infants are reading the article). Disability measures often ignore those in relatively well states. For example, the RAND Health Insurance Study reported that about 80% of the general populations have no dysfunction. Thus, they would estimate that 80% of the population is well. Our method asks about symptoms or problems in addition to behavioral dysfunction (Kaplan and Anderson, 1990). In these studies, only about 12% of the general population report no symptoms on a particular day. In other words, health symptoms or problems are a very common aspect of the human experience. Some might argue that symptoms are unimportant because they are subjective and unobservable. However, symptoms are highly correlated with the demand for medical services, expenditures on health care, and motivations to alter lifestyle. Thus, we feel that the quantification of symptoms is very important.

C. *Utility (Relative Importance)*

Given that various components of morbidity and mortality can be tabulated, it is important to consider their relative importance. For example, it is possible to develop measures that detect very minor symptoms. Yet, because these symptoms are measurable does not necessarily mean they are important. A patient may experience side effects but be willing to tolerate them because the side effects are less important than the probable benefit of consuming the medication. Not all outcomes are equally important. A treatment in which 20 of 100 patients die is not equivalent to one in which 20 of 100 patients develop nausea. An important component of the General Health Policy Model attempts to scale the various health outcomes according to their relative importance. In the preceding example, the relative importance of dying would be weighted more than developing nausea. The weighting is accomplished by rating all states on a continuum ranging from 0 (for death) to 1.0 (for optimum functioning). These ratings are typically provided by independent judges who are representative of the general population. Using this system it is possible to express the relative importance of states in relation to the life-death continuum. A point halfway on the scale (0.5) is regarded as halfway between optimum function and death. The weighting system has been described in several different publications (Kaplan, 1982; Kaplan et al., 1976; Kaplan et al., 1978; Kaplan et al., 1979).

D. *Prognosis*

Another dimension of health status is the duration of a condition. A headache that lasts one hour is not equivalent to a headache that lasts one month. A cough that lasts three days is not equivalent to a cough that lasts three years. In considering the severity of illness, duration of the problem is central. As basic as this concept is, most contemporary models of health outcome measurement completely disregard the duration component. In the General Health Policy Model, the term prognosis refers to the probability of transition among health states over the course of time. In addition to consideration of duration of problems, the model considers the point at which the problem begins. A person may have no symptoms or dysfunctions currently but may have a high probability of health problems in the future. The prognosis component of the model takes these transitions into consideration and applies a discount rate for events that occur in the future.

The Quality of Well-being Scale (QWB) is a method for estimating some components of the general model. The QWB questionnaire categorizes individuals according to functioning and symptoms. Other components of the model are obtained from other data sources (Kaplan and Anderson, 1990).

Applying the Quality of Well-being scale involves several steps. First, patients are classified according to objective levels of functioning.

These levels are represented by scales of mobility, physical activity, and social activity. The dimensions and steps for these levels of functioning are shown in Table I. The reader is cautioned that these steps are not actually the scale, only listings of labels representing the scale steps. Standardized questionnaires have been developed to classify individuals into one of each of these scale steps (Anderson *et al.*, 1986, 1988). In addition to classification into these observable levels of function, individuals are also classified by the one symptom or problem that was most undesirable (see Table II). About half of the population reports at least one symptom on any day. Symptoms may be severe, such as serious chest pain, or minor, such as the inconvenience of taking medication or a prescribed diet for health reasons. The functional classification (Table I) and the accompanying list of symptoms or problems (Table II) was created after extensive reviews of the medical and public health literature (Kaplan *et al.*, 1976). Over the last decade, the function classification system and symptom list were repeatedly shortened until we arrived at the current versions. Various methodological studies on the questionnaire have been conducted (Anderson *et al.*, 1989, 1990, Kaplan *et al.*, 1989). With structured questionnaires an interviewer can obtain classifications on these dimensions in 7 to 15 minutes.

Once observable-behavioral levels of functioning have been classified, a second step is required to place each individual on the 0 to 1.0 scale of wellness. To accomplish this, the observable health states are weighted by "quality" ratings for the desirability of these conditions. Human value studies have been conducted to place to observable states onto a preference continuum with an anchor of 0 for death and 1.0 for completely well. In several studies, random sample of citizens from a metropolitan community evaluated the desirability of over 400 case descriptions. Using these ratings, a preference structure that assigned the weights to each combination of an observable state and a symptom/problem has been developed (Kaplan *et al.*, 1976). Cross validation studies have shown that the model can be used to assign weights to other states of functioning with a high degree of accuracy ($R^2 = 0.96$). The regression weights obtained in these studies are given in Table I and II. Studies have shown that the weights are highly stable over a 1 year period and that they are consistent across diverse groups of raters

(Kaplan *et al.*, 1978). Finally, it is necessary to consider the duration of stay in various health states. For example, one year in a state that has been assigned the weight of 0.5 is equivalent to 0.5 of a Quality Adjusted Life Year. Table I provides an illustrative example of a calculation. Both reliability (Anderson *et al.*, 1989) and validity studies have been published (Kaplan *et al.*, 1976; Kaplan and Anderson, 1990).

The well life expectancy is the current life expectancy adjusted for diminished quality of life associated with dysfunctional states and duration in each state. Using the system, it is possible to simultaneously consider mortality, morbidity, and the preference weights for these observable behavioral states of function. When the proper steps have been followed, the model quantifies the health activity or treatment program in terms of the Quality Adjusted Life Years that it produces or saves. A Quality Adjusted Life Year is defined conceptually as the equivalent of a completely well year of life, or a year of life free of any symptoms, problems, or health related functional limitations.

In summary, this system combines morbidity (the quality of life) and mortality (the duration of life) with prognosis (duration in state). An example of an individual patient might clarify the application of the system. Consider a hypothetical patient with AIDS described in Table III. On the day he was assessed he coughed, wheezed, or was short of breath. He had no limitations in mobility, because he drove his car to the clinic. However, he was in a bed or chair most of the day and performed no major social role. The preference weights associated with the observable state suggests that peers evaluate the state to be about 0.6 on a 0 to 1.0 scale. If the person remains in this state for an entire year, he loses 0.4 well years. If this situation was maintained the course of a decade the person would lose the equivalent of four well year of life.

E. *How This Model Differs from Traditional Conceptualizations*

The two major differences between the GHPM and other approaches to health outcome measurement are: (1) the attempt to express benefits and consequences of health in a common unit known as the well-year or quality-adjusted life year, and (2) emphasis on area under the curve rather than point in time measurement. We argue that the general

TABLE I

Quality of well-being general health policy model: Elements and calculating formulas (function scales, with step definitions and calculating weights)

Step No.	Step Definition	Weight
5	No limitations for health reasons	−0.000
4	Did not drive a car, health related; did not ride in a car as usual for age (younger than 15 yr), health related, *and/or* did not use public transportation, helath related; *or* had or would have used more help than usual for age to use public transportation, health related	−0.062
2	In hospital, health related	−0.090

Physical Activity Scale (PAC)

4	No limitations for health reasons	−0.000
3	In wheelchair, moved or controlled movement of wheelchair without help from someone else; *or* had trouble or did not try to lift, stoop, bend over, or use stairs or inclines, health related; *and/or* limped, used a cane, crutches, or walker, health related; *and/or* had any other physical limitation in walking, or did not try to walk as far as or as fast as others the same age are able, health related	−0.060
1	In wheelchair, did not move or control the movement of wheelchair without help from someone else, *or* in bed, chair, or couch for most or all of the day, health related	−0.077

Social Activity Scale (SAC)

5	No limitations for health reasons	−0.000
4	Limited in other (e.g., recreational) role activity, health related	−0.061
3	Limited in major (primary) role activity, health related	−0.061
2	Performed no major role activity, health related, but did perform self-care activities	−0.106
1	Performed no major role activity, health related, *and* did not perform or had more help than usual in performance of one or more self-care activities, health related	−0.106

TABLE II

Quality of well-being general health policy model: symptom/problem complexes (CPX) with calculating weights

CPX No.	CPX Description	Weights
1	Death (not on respondent's card)	−0.727
2	Loss of consciousness such as seizure (fits), fainting, or coma (out cold or knocked out)	−0.407
3	Burn over large areas of face, body, arms, or legs	−0.387
4	Pain, bleeding, itching, or discharge (drainage) from sexual organs – does not include normal menstrual (monthly) bleeding	−0.349
5	Trouble learning, remembering, or thinking clearly	−0.340
6	Any combination of one or more hands, feet, arms, or legs either missing, deformed (crooked), paralyzed (unable to move), or broken – includes wearing artificial limbs or braces	−0.333
7	Pain, stiffness, weakness, numbness, or other discomfort in chest, stomach (including hernia or rupture), side, neck, back, hips, or any joints or hands, feet, arms, or legs	−0.299
8	Pain, burning, bleeding, itching, or other difficulty with rectum, bowel movements, or urination (passing water)	−0.292
9	Sick or upset stomach, vomiting or loose bowel movement, with or without chills, or arching all over	−0.290
10	General tiredness, weakness, or weight loss	−0.259
11	Cough, wheezing, or shortness of breath, *with* or *without* fever, chills, or arching all over	−0.257
12	Spells of feeling, upset, being depressed, or of crying	−0.257
13	Headache, or dizziness, or ringing in ears, or spells of feeling hot, nervous or shaky	−0.244
14	Burning or itching rash on large areas of face, body, arms, or legs	−0.240
15	Trouble talking, such as lisp, stuttering, hoarseness, or being unable to speak	−0.237
16	Pain or discomfort in one or both eyes (such as burning or itching) or any trouble seeing after correction	−0.230

Table II (continued)

CPX No.	*CPX Description*	Weights
17	Overweight for age and height or skin defect of face, body, arms, or legs, such as scars, pimples, warts, bruises or changes in color	−0.188
18	Pain in ear, tooth, jaw throat, lips, tongue; several missing or crooked permanent teeth – includes wearing bridges or false teeth; stuffy, runny nose; or any trouble hearing – includes wearing a hearing aid	−0.170
19	Taking medication or staying on a prescribed diet for heath reasons	−0.144
20	Wore eyeglasses or contact lenses	−0.101
21	Breathing smog or unpleasant air	−0.101
22	No symptoms or problem (not on respondent's card)	−0.000
23	Standard symptom/problem	−0.257
X24	Trouble Sleeping	−0.257
X25	Intoxication	−0.257
X26	Problemswith sexual interest or performance	−0.257
X27	Excessive worry or anxiety	−0.257

Note: X – Individual weight not available at this time. A standard weight is used instead.

approach to health outcome is, intuitively, what patients and consumers use as a guide. Their physicians may be more directed by a less comprehensive model that considers only a component of health outcome. For example, health care providers might focus on a component of health outcome such as blood pressure. Focusing on a blood pressure might allow the provider to disregard all of the other effects blood pressure management has upon health outcome. Consumers must integrate various sources of information in their decision process. Intuitively they are directed toward maximization of health outcomes. However, sometimes these decision options become overwhelming and the use of a formal model may aid their decision process.

TABLE III

Example calculation for patient with AIDS

Calculating Formulas

Formula 1. Point-in-time well-being score for an individual (W):

$$W = 1 + (1.0 + CPXwt) + (MOBwt) + (PACwt) + (SACwt)$$

where "wt" is the preference-weighted measure for each factor and CPX is Symptom/Problem complex. For example, the W score for a person with the following description profile may be calculated for one day as:

CPX-11	Cough, wheezing or shortness of breath, with or without fever, – chills, or arching all over	0.257
MOB-5	No limitations	−0.000
PAC-1	In bed, chair, or couch for most or all of the day, health related	−0.077
SAC-2	Performed no major role activity, health related, but did perform self-care	−0.061

$$W = 1 + (−0.257) + (−0.000) + (−0.077) + (−0.061) = 0.605$$

Formula 2. Well-years (WY) as an output measure:

$$WY = [\text{No. of persons} \times (CPXwt + MOBwt + PACwt + SACwt) \times Time]$$

A basic objective for most people is to function without symptoms as long as possible. Clearly, early death contradicts this objective. Illness and disability during the interval between birth and death also reduces the total potential health status during a lifetime. Many approaches to health assessment consider only current functioning. We refer to these snapshots of health status as point-in-time measures. The GHPM considers outcome throughout the life cycle. This is what we characterize as the "area under the curve." The more wellness a person experiences throughout the life span, the greater is the area under the curve. Success of interventions is marked by expended area.

The general nature of the health Policy Model leads to some different conclusions than more traditional medical approaches. For example, the traditional medical model focuses on specific diseases and on pathophysiology. Characteristics of illness are quantified according to blood chemistry or in relation to problems in a specific organ system. Often, focus on disease specific outcome measures leads to different conclusions tan those evaluated using a more general outcome measure. For example, studies on the reduction of blood cholesterol have demonstrated reductions in deaths due to coronary heart disease. However,the same studies have failed to demonstrate reductions in total deaths from all causes combined (Lipid Research Clinics coronary Prevention Trial Results, 1984). All studies in the published literature in which patients are assigned to cholesterol lowering through diet or medication, or to a control group, have revealed that reductions in cardiovascular mortality for those in the cholesterol lowering group are compensated for by increase in mortality from other causes (Kaplan, 1984; 1985). A meta-analysis of these studies has demonstrated that the average statistical difference for increase in deaths from non-illness causes (i.e. accidents, murders, etc.) is larger than the average statistical difference for reduction in cardiovascular deaths (Mauldoon *et al.*, 1990).

Similar results have been reported for reductions in cardiovascular deaths attributable to taking aspirin. The disease specific approach focuses on deaths due to myocardial infarction because there is a biological model to describe why aspirin use should reduce heart attacks. Yet, in a controlled experiment in which physician subjects were randomly assigned to take aspirin or placebo, there was no difference in total deaths between the two groups (Kaplan, 1990). Aspirin may reduce the chances of dying from a myocardial infarction, but it does not reduce the chance of dying (Steering Committee of the Physicians' Health Study Research Group, 1988; 1989). The traditional, diagnosis specific, medical model argues that there is a benefit of aspirin because it reduces heart attack, but the general health policy model argues that there is no benefit of aspirin because there is no change in the chances of dying from all causes (Kaplan, 1990).

This same line of reasoning applies to many other areas of health care. Many treatments produce benefits for a specific outcome, but induce side effects that are often neglected in the analysis. Estimates of the benefits of surgery must take into consideration the fact the surgery causes dysfunction through wounds that must heal prior to any realization of the treatment benefits. Further, surgeries often create complications.

The general approach to health status assessment attempts to gain a global picture of the net treatment benefits, taking into consideration both treatment benefits, side effects, and estimates of their relative importance.

Using the information on costs and outcomes, a cost/utility ratio can be formed. This is simply Cost/Well-years.

The model for point in time with Quality of Well-being is:

QWB = 1   – (observed morbidity × morbidity weight)
         – (observed physical activity × physical activity weight)
         – (observed social activity and social activity weight)
         – (observed symptom/problem × symptom/problem weight).

Consider, for example, a person who is in an objective state of functioning that is rated by community peers as 0.5 on a 0 to 1.0 scale. If the person remains in the state for one year they have lost the equivalent of 1/2 of one year of life. So, for example, a person limited in activities who requires a cane or walker to get around the community might be hypothetically at 0.50. Over the course of an entire year, he or she would lose the equivalent of one year of life. A person who has the flu may also get 0.50, but the illness might only last three days. Thus, the total loss in well-years might be $3/365 \times 0.50 = 0.004$ well-years.

The cost/utility ratio is defined as:

$$\frac{Cw - Cwo}{Ww - Wwo}$$

Where   Cw is the cost with the treatment or program
           Cwo is the cost without the treatment or program
           Ww is the well years with the treatment or program
           Wwo is the well years of life without the treatment or program

Using the cost/well year ratio it is possible to rank order various programs. Typically, potential programs are rank-ordered by how much they return for the invested dollar. Interpretation of a rank order list must take available resources into consideration. If enough resources are available, all services can be covered. However, if resources are restricted, funding programs according to the ordering on the list will provide the most health to the population given that resources are restricted.

Another may to evaluate outcomes is within "policy space." Various approaches to cost/benefit and cost/utility analysis occasionally produce different results. The output for cost/benefit analysis is in monetary terms – a program that produces cost savings. Cost/utility analysis focuses on the cost to produce a well-year of life. Anderson *et al.* (1986) integrated the concepts of well-years and net dollars returned within a common framework. This was accomplished by creating a two-dimensional policy space as illustrated in Fig. 1. The x-axis in the figure represents net dollars returned per person. Returns are defined as benefits minus costs in dollar units. The y-axis displays well-year lost or gained through a particular treatment program, clinical intervention, or policy change.

The right half of the plane would be used a represent programs in which benefits exceed costs, while the left half would display situations in which costs exceed benefits. The upper half of the figure displays outcomes that have positive health effects in terms of QALYs. Those in the bottom half of the figure would be used to represent negative health outcomes in QALY units.

The two dimensional space yields four quadrants. One quadrant, the lower left, represents unsuitable alternatives. In these cases, dollars are being spent and negative health consequences occur. Administration of a uniformly toxic treatment might be represented by this quadrant. The upper right quadrant represents the most attractive alternatives. Here, QALY health benefits are gained and there are also economic benefits. Prevention of early heart disease might be an example. The upper left quadrant shows QALY gains, but with more significant costs associated with these improvements. Transplantation surgery for the elderly might be described by this quadrant. Here, there are significant health benefits, but the recipients may not return to the productive economic sector.

The lower right quadrant represents another level of economic trade-off. Here, society may be willing to sacrifice some health benefits in exchange for cost savings. Anderson and colleagues suggested that

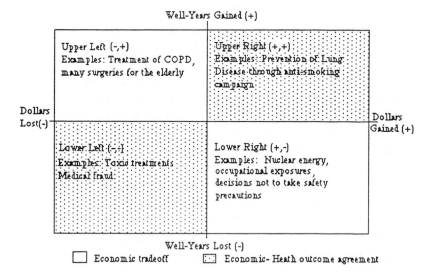

Fig. 1. A two-dimensional policy space. The x-axis in the figure represents net dollars returned per person. Returns are defined as benefits minus costs in dollar units. The y-axis displays QALY lost or gained through a particular treatment program, clinical intervention, or policy change.

these tradeoffs may be common in studies involving nuclear power, pollution control, occupational, environmental, and consumer product safety, highway speed limits, etc.

APPLICATIONS OF THE MODEL

The notion that we should invest in health services that make people well seems straight forward. Yet, the application of this model is difficult. The major problem is that different programs in health care have different objectives. Some health care providers are trying to reduce the infant mortality rate. Rheumatologists strive to make their patients more functional while primary care providers often focus on shortening the cycle of acute illness. All of these providers are attempting to improve the health of their patients. However, they all measure health in

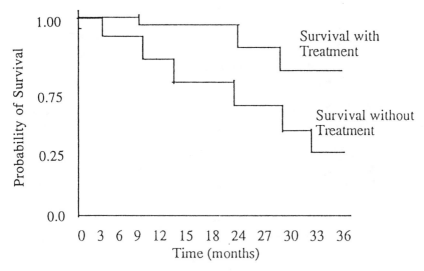

Fig. 2.   A common comparison in survival analysis. The upper curve describes the probability of living to various ages, given that treatment is received. The lower curve describes the probability of living to these same ages in the absence of treatment. The difference in the area between the curves describes the impact of the intervention.

different ways, Comparing the productivity of a rheumatologist versus an oncologist may be like comparing apples to oranges.

The diversity of outcomes in health care has led many analysts to focus on the simplest common ground. Typically, that is mortality or life expectancy. When mortality is studied, those who are alive are statistically coded as 1.0 while those who are dead are statistically coded as 0.0. Mortality allows the comparison between different diseases. For example, we can state the life expectancy for those who will eventually die of heart disease and compare it to the life expectancy to those who eventually die of cancer. The difficulty is that everyone who remains alive is given the same score. A person confined to bed with an irreversible coma is alive and is counted the same as someone who is actively playing volley ball at a picnic. One purpose of the Quality of Well-being scale is to quantify levels of wellness on the continuum between death and optimum function. Figure 2 shows a common comparison in survival

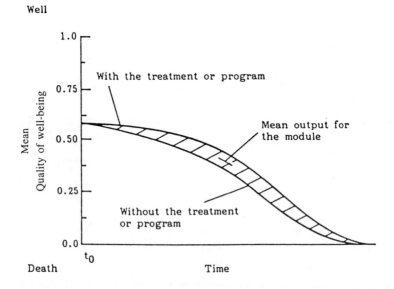

Fig. 3.   Survival analysis that adjusts for quality of life. In other words, this figure rates the degree of dysfunction along this scale. The difference in the ares between the curves in represents adjusted years of life.

analysis. The upper curve describes the probability of living to various ages, given that treatment is received. The lower curve describes the probability of living to these same ages in the absence of treatment. The difference in the area between the curves describes the impact of the intervention. Figure 3 shows a similar survival analysis that adjusts for quality of life. In other words, this figure rates the degree of dysfunction along this scale. The difference in the areas between the curves in Fig. 3 represents quality adjusted years of life. In other words, this is a survival analysis that adjusts for quality of life.

EXAMPLES OF CLINICAL PROBLEMS

There is growing pressure to make difficult health resources decisions. For example, the Department of Veteran Affairs (DVA) runs the largest chain of hospitals in the United States. These DVA medical centers once enjoyed substantial freedom in medication choices. Recently, however, budgets in the DVA have been constrained. The pharmacies have been asked to review alternatives and make formulary decisions about which products should be kept in stock. In response, the hospitals appointed formulary committees to help make these difficult decisions. Similar formulary decision challenges began in several other countries, including Australia and Canada (Province of Ontario). One of the major difficulties is that the committees had very little data to guide their decisions. Further, the committees typically included physicians from competing medical specialties who are unable to find a common language that could be used to compare the different treatment alternatives. One application of the General Health Policy model is to help with this type of decision.

Other applications of the model are more clinical. Treatments have side effects and they have benefits. When outcome measures are highly focused, researchers may measure positive effects but ignore the negative. For example, treatments for hypertension have typically been evaluated in terms of reductions in blood pressure. However, these same treatments also produce headaches, dizziness, and impotence in males. For many years, researchers never even bothered to evaluate these side effects. Once documentation of side effects began, we were left with the difficult problem of knowing that the drugs did some good and some harm. Despite side effects, many drugs are worth using because the benefits outweigh the consequences. The challenge is to evaluate all the benefits and all the side effects and come to a comprehensive evaluation of treatment value. This chapter gives some examples of GHPM applications relevant to these different problems. The General Health Policy Model has now been used for a variety of different purpose. It is not possible to review all of these applications here. Instead, some selected applications of the model will be presented.

It is important to emphasize that the QWB scale is the measurement system for a General Health Policy Model. Ultimately, we hope that clinical trials will incorporate these measures so the estimates of treatment effects can be obtained in well-year units. Many of the analyses presented in this section depend upon estimates of QWB scores rather than the actual measurements but are presented to emphasize the potential for utilizing quality of life measures for policy studies.

THE TIGHT CONTROL OF INSULIN-DEPENDENT DIABETES MELLITUS

Several studies have suggested that the degree of hyperglycemia is associated with the long term risk of diabetic complications (Tchobroutsky, 1978). In addition to mortality, diabetes may be associated with poor outcomes in a variety of organ systems. For example, poor control might lead to differential rates of retinopathy, kidney failure, and foot infections. However, until recently, there was no strong experimental evidence confirming that reduction in blood sugar lead to a parallel reduction in diabetic complications. The question of tight control of diabetes was considered important enough for the US National Institutes of Health to conduct a prospective clinical trial to evaluate the benefits to tight control versus ordinary care. The trial, known as the Diabetes Control and Complications Trial (DCCT) included approximately 1 400 subjects. The study cost over $200 million and was halted before the planned ten year finish date because the results were encouraging. Despite the attractiveness of this well controlled clinical trial, the DCCT still left many important questions about the treatment of diabetes unanswered (Lasker, 1993).

The DCCT focused on a single intervention (intensive control of diabetes) and considered as endpoints only a single group of established physiological measures. In particular, they measured micro vascular complications and placed greatest emphasis in retinopathy. The results of the study did indicate small but significant reductions in the chances of developing micro vascular and neurologic complications among those randomly assigned to intensive insulin therapy (DCCT, 1993). However, the trail did not measure the significant financial and personal costs of using this intensive therapy.

A comprehensive evaluation of diabetes treatment may require measures that capture all of the different effects of the illness and its treatment. Some patients may have foot infections that result in amputations, while others have eye problems that result in blindness. One purpose of the General Health Policy Model is to aggregate these outcomes with death to provide a single expression of the impact of poor control. Diabetic coma receives a score of approximately 0.32 on the QWB while vision impairment that interferes with driving a car and work, but does not interfere with self-care might receive score of 0.61. This tells us that two days of diabetic coma add up to less than one day of vision impairment. However, treatment that eliminates diabetic coma (averaged across the duration of the coma) might be considered more valuable than one that reduces vision impairment. The objective is to eliminate any sort of impairment. However, the QWB does provide for some weighting of the very different outcomes assessed in the study.

The system also includes the capability of expressing side-effects and benefits of treatments in the same unit. For example, suppose that the treatment reduces the probability of retinopathy by 25%. We will assume that 40% of the patients will eventually get serious retinopathy (Klein and Klein, 1985). Suppose further that the retinopathy begins at age 55 and continues until death at an average age of 75. The weight associated with blindness or serious vision impairment might be 0.5. The GHPM calculations suggest that the chances of developing serious retinopathy (0.4) multiplied by average decrease in well-being by 20 years and then multiplied by the times (0.5) reduction in severity resulting from treatment (0.25) would equal 1.0 well-year. In other words, the improved treatment of diabetes might add up to the equivalent of one healthy year of life expectancy.

Now, we must consider the consequences or side effects of tight control. For the sake of argument, assume that the intensive treatment begins at age 30. One third of the patients experience nausea and weakness associated with tight control on half of the days. So, let us assume that the duration is $75 - 30 = 45$ years, divided by the number of days in which there are symptoms, $0.5 \times 45 = 22.5$ years multiplied by the weight associated with the symptom of sick or upset stomach which is 0.75. The net side effects occur for 0.33 of all patients × 22.5 years × 0.25 average decrease in QWB = 1.87 years. In this example the side effects might cause a loss of the equivalent of 1.87 years while the benefits are about 1.0 years. However, the benefits for other aspects of treatment must also be considered. So, for example, we would also consider the altered probability of kidney disease, heart disease, etc. With these added in, the benefits would most likely outweigh the side effects. However, intensive insulin therapy also has financial and human costs. For example, intensive therapy may cost between $8 and $10 thousand (US) per year in comparison to usual care. Further, there may be additional burdens of inconvenience that are not directly measured through symptoms.

Ultimately, the net effects of a treatment are expressed in these Well-year or QALY units. The next question concerns determination of the costs to produce a quality adjusted or well year unit, from which comparison health care programs with very different specific objectives may be made. These calculations have been completed for several treatments, including medication for arthritis.

AURANOFIN TREATMENT FOR PATIENTS WITH RHEUMATOID ARTHRITIS

Clinical trials for treatments of rheumatoid arthritis have considered a wide variety of end points. The traditional approach has been to review clinical outcomes such as degree of synovitis. This is typically assessed through tender or swollen joints, grip strength, time to walk 40 feet, or duration of stiffness upon rising in the morning. At an international conference on outcome measurement in arthritis, it was suggested that comprehensive assessments of quality of life outcomes were highly desirable (Bombardier et al., 1982). In one clinical trial involving 14 centers, more than 300 patients were randomly assigned to therapy with oral gold (auranofin) or a placebo. A wide variety of traditional and non-traditional measures were used to assess outcome, and among the non-traditional measures was the QWB Scale. The outcome using the QWB is shown graphically in Fig. 4. There was

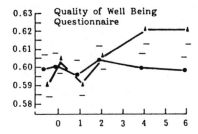

Fig. 4. The outcome of auranofin study using the QWB.

essentially no change in QWB function for the placebo group while the group receiving auranofin showed a mean improvement of 0.023. This difference was statistically significant beyond the 0.005 level. Auranofin does not reach pharmacologically effective levels in blood until it has been used for about two months. It is interesting that QWB scores for the treatment and placebo groups begin to diverge at about two months. Considering the many measures used in the trial, the percentage of variance accounted for with the QWB measure was among the very most significant (see Fig. 5). Outcomes measured using traditional, clinical measures, such as the 50-foot walk and duration of morning stiffness were not statistically significant, although they did favor the auranofin group. In addition, simple self ratings by both patients and physicians failed to detect the significant effect. However, a significant network of associations emerged suggesting that the QWB was associated with other similar measures of general function (Bombardier *et al.*, 1986).

It is important to consider the clinical importance of a difference of 0.023. Although this appears to be a small number, the QWB provides a direct translation into clinically meaningful units. A difference of 0.023 translates into 2.3 Quality Adjusted Life Years for each 100 patients who maintain the difference for 1 year. Also, although 0.023 appears to be a small change, the entire continuum from death to optimal health is represented on the 0 to 1.0 scale. The differences observed in the auranofin trial are quite respectable in comparison to those obtained through other medical treatments.

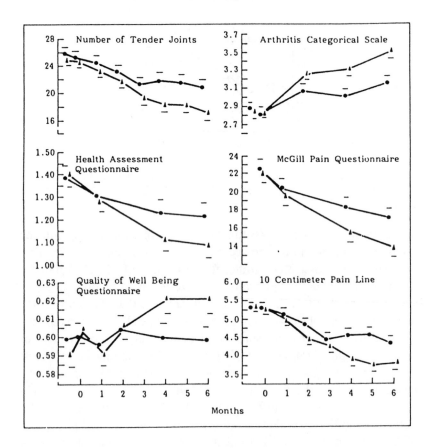

Fig. 5.   Among the many measures used in the trial, the percentage of variance accounted for with the QWB measure was among the very most significant (From Bombardier *et al.* 1986, reproduced with permission).

One of the most important aspects of the QWB is its capability of quantifying side effects as well as benefits. Many of the specific scales used for the auranofin trial were not capable of detecting the general effect of the intervention upon health status. Yet, gold preparations are known to cause significant adverse effects including diarrhea, headache, rashes, digestive problems, and abdominal pain. In fact, 59%

of the auranofin treated patients experienced diarrhea at some point in comparison to 19% of the placebo treated group. The General Health Policy Model allowed these side effects to be integrated with benefits in order to provide a comprehensive expression on net treatment efficacy. Thompson and colleagues (1988) evaluated the cost/utility of auranofin treatment. In comparison to control subjects, the costs associated with auranofin treatment were $788 per patient. The investigators estimated the cost/utility of auranofin therapy at just more than $10 000 US dollars per well year of life. This compares quite favorably to many alternatives in health care.

THE ACQUIRED IMMUNODEFICIENCY SYNDROME (AIDS)

The Acquired Immune Deficiency syndrome (AIDS), resulting from infection with the human immunodeficiency virus (HIV) represents one of the most important threats to the world population in the 1990's. The Centers for Disease Control estimates that between one and two million Americans are currently infected with HIV (Centers for Disease Control, 1991). The World Health Organization (1993) estimates that over 13 million people had been infected with HIV by 1993 and projections suggest that the pandemic continues to be out of control.

In addition to opportunistic infections and malignancies which define AIDS, HIV infection may cause a broad range of disease. These conditions include persistent lymphadenopathy, thrombocytopenia, immune complex disease, wasting, various constitutional symptoms, and HIV neurologic disease. The impact of HIV infection on functioning is equally diverse. For example, HIV infection may result in fatigue, arthritis, blindness, memory loss, or paraplegia. Treatments for HIV infection should be designed to prevent early mortality and to reduce morbidity during periods before death. The diverse impacts of both HIV disease and its treatment require a general approach to assessment.

There have been several previous attempts to evaluate quality of life in HIV infected patients. However, most of these have focused on psychological outcomes. Few studies have attempted to characterize the health status and economic impacts of HIV infection and we are aware of only a few studies that have applied general health-related quality of life scales.

Since September 1987, AZT has been available by prescription to treat patients with advanced HIV infection. This decision was based on the encouraging results of early clinical trials. In the multicenter phase II AZT trial, 19 of 137 placebo recipients died as compared to 1 of 145 AZT recipients. The incidence of opportunistic infections was also significantly reduced among AZT recipients. Thus, in certain groups of patients, AZT may profoundly lower both mortality and morbidity (Fischl *et al.*, 1987). However, serious side effects are frequently associated with AZT, including anemia, neutropenia, nausea, myalgia, insomnia, and severe headache. Nearly one third (31%) of patients who received AZT required blood transfusions for anemia (Richman *et al.*, 1987).

In the San Diego arm of the multicenter AZT trial, Wu *et al.* obtained outcome data using the QWB and the Karnofsky Performance Status measure (Wu *et al.*, 1990). The participants in the study were 31 patients (27 male, 4 female) with a clinical diagnosis of either AIDS or severe AIDS Related Complex (ARC). They were randomly assigned to receive AZT treatment or placebo and were evaluated using the QWB before beginning the trial and at eight follow-up visits over the next 52 weeks. The value of the treatment was estimated using the repeated measures analysis of variance (calculated using a general linear model).

The patients were divided into those with CD4 cell (also known as T_4 lymphocytes or T-helper cell) counts less than or greater than $100 \times 10^9 L$. Patients in both groups were comparable at baseline with regard to age, CD4 group, sex, diagnosis (AIDS or ARC), Karnofsky score, and QWB (*t*-test and chi-square, $p > 0.15$). In fact, mean initial CD4 count was significantly higher in the AZT group ($t < 0.03$).

For the QWB measure, the repeated measures ANOVA showed a significant effect of time and an interaction between group and time of testing. This interaction, illustrated in Fig. 6, is the crucial component in evaluating treatment effectiveness. It suggests that there was a differential rate of change between AZT treated and control groups. As Fig. 6 demonstrates, QWB scores remained relatively constant over the course of time for the AZT group, while they declined substantially for the placebo group.

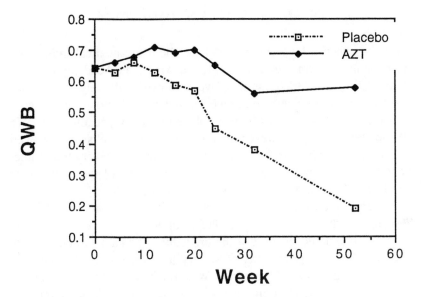

Fig. 6. Significant effect of time and an interaction between group and time of testing in the AZT trial. There was a different rate of change between AZT treated and control groups: QWB scores remained relatively constant over the course of time for the AZT group, while they declined substantially for the placebo group.

These results suggest that the QWB can detect strong treatment effects associated with AZT treatment. One advantage of the QWB system is that it allows the expression of program benefits in terms of QALY units and the comparison of treatment alternatives that are very different from one another. In the AZT trial, the placebo-treated group experienced substantial mortality and greater morbidity than the AZT group. Neither measures of mortality alone, nor of morbidity alone, were capable of detecting the potent treatment effect of this medication, as could the QWB. Further, the comprehensive measure takes the side-effects of AZT into account and expresses outcome as the net benefits minus adverse effects (Kaplan, 1991).

THE NEONATAL CIRCUMCISION CONTROVERSY

There has been a long standing debate about the medical indications for neonatal circumcision. In 1971, the American Academy of Pediatrics (1971) concluded that there were no medically valid reasons for performing circumcisions on newborn males. This position was confirmed by the American College of Obstetrics and Gynecology in 1978 (Wallerstein, 1985). However, an important paper by Wiswell (Wiswell and Roscelli, 1986) suggested a tenfold increase in urinary tract infections for uncircumcised male infants. As a results of these data, new questions about an old controversy began to arise.

Recently a cost/utility analysis was performed in order to estimate the total health effects and the total costs of neonatal circumcision. The analysis considered the cost of the procedure, the pain associated with the procedure, the probability of urinary tract infections, and the risks of developing cancer of the penis. With the base assumptions, the net discounted lifetime US dollar costs associated with neonatal circumcision were relatively low ($102 US/person). However, the discounted lifetime health costs were also quite low. Under the base assumptions, the expected health benefit is about 14 hours of well-life expectancy.

In cases such as the evaluation of neonatal circumcision, it is unlikely that a true randomized trial will ever be conducted. Therefore, the analysis typically consider outcomes under a variety of circumstances. However we are often uncertain about the accuracy of these assumptions. In order to deal with the uncertainty, the assumptions are varied. In the circumcision example, the base analysis assumed that the probability of developing cancer if uncircumcised is 0.0001 while the probability for those who are circumcised is essentially 0.000. In the sensitivity analysis, it was assumed that the probability of developing cancer if uncircumcised is more severe. For example, it may be as high as 1/600 or 0.00167. The development of cancer may also have important cost implication. In the base case it was assumed that the work up and treatment costs would be $25 000. The sensitivity analysis considered a lower estimate of $10 000 and a higher estimate of $100 000. Many variables are considered in the sensitivity analyses. For example, the cost of the procedure is considered to be $150 US dollars in the base case while in the sensitivity analysis a lower cost of $50 was also included. The traditional method for comparing a value to be received in the future (e.g. medical expenses averted) with a value to be given at the present time (in this case the cost of the circumcision) is discounting. With the aim of looking at future gains and comparing them with the amount of money currently at hand, compound discount-rate multipliers are typically included in the analysis. In this analysis discount rates in the base case were 5% while a discount rate of 0% was considered for the sensitivity analysis. The discount rate multipliers were also used with the number of well-years produced.

Under the base case assumptions, the costs of routine neonatal circumcision are $102 451 and the effects are an average loss of 1.61 Well-years. Any program that damages health as a function of treatment is not advisable. However, under some assumptions, the analysis suggests more benefits. For example, in the case that a patient needs a second circumcision and experiences symptoms for 120 days prior to the second operation, the cost/utility ratio is $18 463/well year. If the cost of the later circumcision is $5 000 US dollars, than the cost/utility ratio becomes $45 673/well year. The base case assumes that the cost of circumcision is $150 US dollars. Although the cost/utility of the procedure in the base case is questionable, reducing the cost of the procedure to $50 US dollars makes the intervention look more worthwhile at $9 054/well year. The advantage is because money is saved, not because better health is achieved. Overall, the financial and medical advantages of neonatal circumcision cancel each other out. In this case cost/utility analysis helped clarify that the issue is not one of economics or medical outcome. Instead, the debate must be focused on personal preference and social custom (Gamiats *et al.*, 1991).

TOBACCO TAX

The use of tobacco products, and particularly cigarette smoking, is a widespread problem in nearly all countries of the world. In the United States, there are an estimated 56 million smokers. In California alone, the $0.25 per pack tax raises nearly 600 million dollars per year. Substantial evidence reported by the Surgeon General (1989) suggests that cigarette smoking causes an excessive number of preventable deaths. Although cigarette smoking has declined in the United Sates and the United Kingdom within recent years, the worldwide trend is toward increased use of tobacco products. Richard Peto and colleagues, through the World Health Organization, projects that, worldwide, there will be 10 million tobacco related deaths per year by the Year 2010 (Peto *et al.*, 1992). The importance of the cigarette smoking problem is summarized in recent data reported by McGinnis and Foege (1993). Their calculations suggest that about 25 000 annual deaths in the US can be attributed to motor vehicle crashes, and about 20 000 deaths can be attributed to illicit drug use. In contrast, there are about 400 000 deaths associated with tobacco use. That is 20 times the number associated with drug use and 16 times the number associated with auto crashes. The public is very concerned about dramatic causes of death such as being killed by an accident at work, or being killed by a drunk driver. However, for each person killed by a drunk driver, nearly 74 active smokers die prematurely (see Fig. 7).

There are many different approaches to the reduction of cigarette smoking. One of the most effective ways to control cigarette use is to increase the price of these products. Economists use the term elasticity to refer to changes in demand that occur as a function a price. Although there has been some debate about whether or not the demand for tobacco products is "elastic," the emerging consensus is that a significant proportion of the variation in tobacco use *is* responsive to price.

Figure 8 shows the relationship between price per pack of cigarettes and cigarettes consumed in 22 European countries. As the figure shows, there is a rough linear relationship between price and consumption. Countries charging more per pack tend to have lower rates of cigarette smoking, while countries charging less per pack tend to have higher rates. Norway, for example, with a $4.17 per pack charge which includes $2.71 in tax, has evolved the lowest smoking rate in Europe (World Health Organization, 1987). However, these data are a snapshot of a particular point is time, and do not address how the *introduction* of a tax affects consumption. This is being examined in our evaluation of the California tax. Figure 9 shows the smoking prevalence trends among

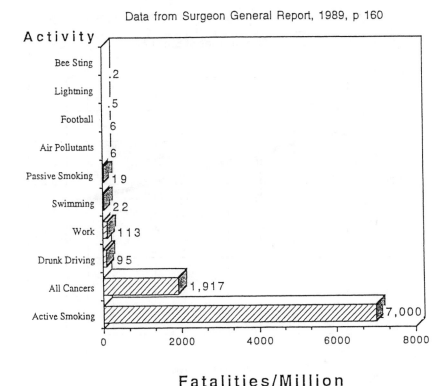

Fig. 7.   Fatalities in the US population associated with various causes (based on data from the US Surgeon General's report).

Californians age 20 years and older before and after the introduction of the $0.25 tax. Data for this analysis come from the US National Health Interview Survey, the Current Population Survey, the Behavioral Risk Factor Survey, and our California Tobacco Survey. Combining these sources, we estimate that prior to the tax, the prevalence of smoking was declining at a rate of 0.70 percent per year. Since the introduction of the tax, the rate of decline has accelerated to 1.27 percent per year. Other evidence from the study indicates that price is a factor in consumption

Price of cigarettes and cigarette consumption per adult per
year.
22 countries of Europe

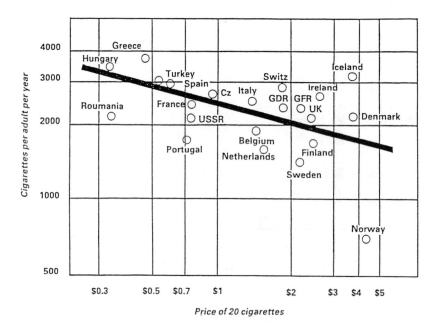

Fig. 8. The relationship between price per pack of cigarettes and cigarettes consumed
among 22 European countries (Source: World Health Organization, 1987).

decisions. For example, the change in the rate of decline is significantly
greater for socioeconomically disadvantaged groups.

The motivation for health care reform is to save lives and improve
the public health. It is assumed that the best way to accomplish this goal
is to invest in medical care. However, a significant tobacco excise tax
will enhance health status while raising revenue. In order to evaluate the
impact of tobacco taxes, we developed a series of computer simulations.
Employing a series of different assumptions to estimate the impact of
increasing the tobacco tax, under the model presented here, we assumed
an elasticity (a change in the percentage demand divided by the change

Smoking Prevalence Among Californians Age 20 and Older

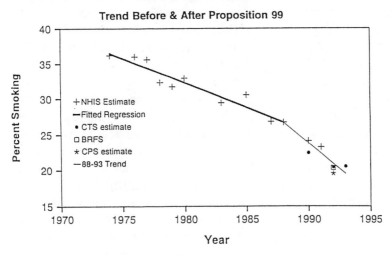

Source: NHIS 1974-1991; CTS 1990, 1992, 1993; BRFS 1992; CPS 1992

Fig. 9. Prevalence of cigarette smoking among adults in California before and after the introduction at the 1989 $0.25 per pack tobacco tax (From Pierce *et al.*, 1993, public domain).

in the percentage price) of −0.26. The assumption used here suggests, for example, that if there is a 20% increase in price, there will be approximately a 5% decrease in demand. The −0.26 value was taken from the estimates of price elasticity for smokers of all ages as reported in the US Surgeon General's report in 1989. These estimates are based on three studies by Lewit and Coate (1983). The elasticity estimate is among the most conservative reported in the literature.

In one analysis that we conducted, using a method called a Monte Carlo simulation, we assumed that there are about 56 million smokers in the US and that one in four of these smokers will eventually die of a tobacco related disease, and a tax increase of 20% (considerably less than that proposed in the US). Using a computer to generate data under various assumptions, this analysis considers the expected change in life expectancy for smokers and builds in a model of reduced quality of life for smokers beginning at age 50. These methods combine death and reduced life quality into a single index know as the Quality Adjusted Life Year (QALY). A death premature by one year is represented by the loss of one QALY. A year of life in which quality is reduced by one half because of a disease, is represented by the lose of 0.50 QALYs. The prevalence rate for reduced life expectancy and dysfunction are based on national estimates from the Health Interview Survey. According to the analysis, there is a 50% chance that we could save 6.4 million Quality-Adjusted Life Years in the US by increasing tobacco taxes by 20%. The model shows that there is a 90% chance of saving about three million Quality-Adjusted Life years (see Fig. 10). To put these figure into perspective, the total annual health effect of arthritis is estimated to cost society 5 million equivalents of Quality-Adjusted Life Years, while the impact of homicide is about 1.5 million years. In other words, the public health benefits of an increased tobacco tax may well exceed the benefit of having a whole year without arthritis or of eliminating our epidemic of homicide for one year. We know of no other health services that can improve the public health to the extent estimated to be attributable to an increased tobacco tax (Kaplan, 1993).

The tax would benefit society by reducing the burden of disease and disability and may directly benefit smokers by providing incentives to quit early. The losers in this scheme would be smokers who choose to continue their habit, and the tobacco industry. However, data from our California surveys indicate that the majority of smokers want to quit and about 50% of smokers make an active attempt to quit each year (Pierce *et al.*, 1993).

Overall, the analysis suggests that there is a public health advantage to raising tobacco taxes. Similar conclusions have been reached by other researchers (Warner, 1986). It is important to emphasize that this is among several simulations we have conducted. However, even under the most conservative assumptions, the model shows that increased tobacco taxes will improve health more than many accepted medical care programs.

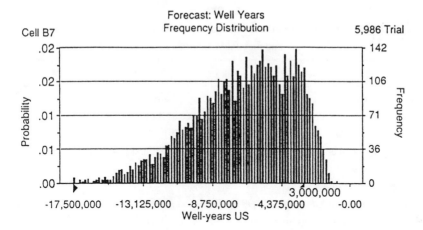

Fig. 10.   Estimated number of quality adjusted life years saved by a 20% increase in tobacco tax.

COMPARISONS ACROSS DIFFERENT PROGRAMS

Table IV summarizes the cost/well-year of life estimated for several medical, surgical, and preventive interventions. Using this system we can begin to rank order the value for money for many interventions in health care. Among programs that have been analyzed, the most cost/effective option in not a medical procedure. Instead, it is a program that requires children to be in infant seats and adults to be in seat belts. Public health programs, such as thyroid disease screening programs (T4), PKU screening, and screening for high blood pressure, all compete very favorably. However, some screening programs such as mammography are less cost/effective than other options. Some surgical options used for rescue, including coronary artery bypass surgery for one vessel disease, produce less health for the dollar invested. Tables, such as IV depend upon many assumption and improved analysis is required before we can feel assured that the comparisons are correct. However, enough data are accumulating to begin making these comparisons.

TABLE IV

Summary of cost/well-year estimates for selected medical, surgical,
and preventive interventions[a]

Program	Reference	Cost/Well-Year
Seat belt laws	Kaplan (1988)	0
Ante-partum and anti-D injection[b]	Torrance & Zipursky (1984)	1,543
Pneumonococcal vaccine for the elderly	OTA (1979)	1,765
Post-partum and anti-D injection[b]	Torrance & Zipursky (1977)	2,109
Coronary artery bypass surgery for left main coronary	Weinstein (1982)	4,922
Neonatal intensive care, 1,000–14,999 g	Boyle et al. (1983)	5,473
Smoking cessation counseling	Schulman (1991)	6,463
T4 (thyroid) screening	Epstein et al. (1981)	7,595
PKU screening[c]	Bush et al. (1973)	8,498
Treatment of severe hypertension (diastolic > 105 mm Hg) in males age 40	Stason & Weinstein (1977)	10,896
Oral gold in rheumatoid arthritis	Thompson et al. (1987)	12,059
Dapsone for prophylaxis for PCP pneumonia[d]	Freedberg (1991)	13,400
Treatment of mild hypertension (diastolic 95–104 mm Hg) in males age 40	Weinstein & Stason (1976)	22,197
Oat bran for high cholesterol	Kinosian et al. (1988)	22,910
Rehabilitation in COPD[e]	Toevs et al. (1984)	28,320
Estrogen therapy for postmenopausal symptoms in women without a prior hysterectomy	Weinstein (1980)	32,057
Neonatal intensive care, 500–999 g	Boyle et al. (1983)	38,531
CABG (surgery) 2-vessel disease[f]	Weinstein & Stason (1982)	39,770
Hospital hemodialysis	Churchill et al. (1984)	40,200
Coronary artery bypass surgery for single-vessel disease with moderately severe occlusion	Weinstein (1981)	42,195

Table IV (continued)

Program	Reference	Cost/Well-Year
School tuberculin testing program	Bush *et al.* (1972)	43,250
Continuous ambulatory peritoneal dialysis	Churchill *et al.* (1984)	54,460
Cholestipol for high cholesterol	Kinosian *et al.* (1988)	92,467
Cholestyramine for high cholesterol	Kinosian *et al.* (1988)	153,105
Screening mammography	Eddy (1990)	167,850
Total hip replacement	Liang (1987)	293,029
CABG (surgery) 1-vessel heart disease[f]	Weinstein & Stason (1982)	662,835
Aerosolized pentamidine for prophylaxis of PCP pneumonia[d]	Freedberg (1991)	756,000

[a] All estimates adjusted to 1991 U.S. dollars, [b] treatment for Rh immunization;
[c] PKU, phenylketonuria; [d] PCP, pneumocystic carinii pneumonia;
[e] COPD, chronic obstructive pulmonary disease;
[f] CABG, coronary artery bypass graft.

From Kaplan, 1993

SUMMARY

This chapter summarizes some of our current thinking on the potential for a general health policy model. We believe the system can be used as an aid for understanding clinical and public health problems. Several examples of the use of the QWB in clinical decision making are offered. Current research is often divided between measurement studies and policy analysis. The General Health Policy Model includes the measurement system described here. When taken in clinical studies, QWB measurements can be used directly in policy analysis. However, few clinical studies have taken QWB measures directly. The examples summarized in this chapter show how programs with very different objectives can be compared directly with one another.

NOTES

Portions of this chapter were adapted from Kaplan, R M (1993) *The Hippocratic Predicament: Affordability, Access and Accountability in American Medicine*. San Diego: Academic Press and from Kaplan, R. M., Anderson, J. P., & Ganiats, T. G. (1993) The quality of well-being scale: rationale for a single quality of life index. In S. R. Walker & R. M. Rosser (eds) *Qualit of life assessment: Key issues in the 1990s*. London: Kluwer Academic Publishers, pp. 65–94.

Supported in part by grants from the California Policy Seminar and The National Institutes of Health and Gant P60 AR 40770 from the National Institute of Arthritis, Musculoskeletal, and Skin Diseases of the National Institutes of Health.

REFERENCES

American Academy of Pediatrics, Committee on Fetus and Newborn: 1991, Hospital Care of Newborn Infants 5th ed. (American Academy of Pediatrics, Winston, IL).

Anderson J. P., J. W. Bush and C. C. Berry: 1986, 'Classifying function for health outcome and quality-of-life evaluation. Self versus individual models', Medical Care 24, pp. 454–469.

Anderson, J. P., J. W. Bush, M. Chen and D. Dolenc: 1986, 'Policy space areas and properties of BCU analysis', Journal of the American Medical Associated 255, pp. 794–795.

Anderson, J. P., R. M. Kaplan and M. BeBon: 1989, 'Comparison of responses to similar questions in health surveys', in F. Fowler (ed.), Health Survey Research Methods (National Center for Health Statistics, Washington, DC), pp. 13–21.

Anderson, J. P., R. M. Kaplan, C. C. Berry, J. W. Bush and R. G. Rumbaut: 1989, 'Interday reliability of function assessment for a health status measure: The quality of well-being scale', Medical Care 27, pp. 1076–1084.

Ballugooie, E. *et al.*: 1983, 'Rapid deterioration of diabetic retinopathy during treatment with continuous subcutaneous insulin infusion', Diabetes Care 7, pp. 236–242.

Bombardier, C., J. Ware and I. J. Russell *et al.*: 1986, 'Auranofin therapy and quality of life for patients with rheumatoid arthritis: Results of a multicenter trial', American Journal of Medicine 81, pp. 565–578.

Brook, R. H. and K. Lohr: 1986, 'Will we need to ration effective health care?', issues in Science and Technology 3, pp. 68–77.

Centers for Disease Control: 1991, 'Mortality attributable to HIV infection/AIDS United States 1981–1990', Morbidity and Mortality Weekly Report 40(3), p. 41.

Diabetes Control and Complications Group: 1993, 'The effect of intensive treatment of diabetes on the development and progression of long-term complications in insulin-dependent diabetes mellitus. The Diabetes Control and Complications Trial Research Group', New England Journal of Medicine 329, pp. 977–986.

Fischl, M. A., D. D. Richman and M. H. Grieco *et al.*: 1987, 'The efficiency of azidothymidine (AZT) in the treatment of patients with AIDS and AIDS-related complex: A double-blind, placebo-controlled trial', New England Journal of Medicine 317, pp. 185–191.

Ganiats, T. G., J. D. C. Humphrey, H. L. Tares and R. M. Kaplan: 1991, 'Routine neonatal circumcision: A cost-utility analysis', Medical Decision Making 11, pp. 282–293.

Hu, T., J. Bai, T. E. Keeler and P. G. Barnett: 1991, 'The impact of a large tax increase on cigarette consumption: The case of California', Unpublished Manuscript, School of Public Health, University of California, Berkeley.

Kaplan R. M.: 1984, 'The connection between clinical health promotion and health status: A critical review', American Psychologist 39, pp. 755–765.

Kaplan R. M.: 1985, 'Behavioral epidemiology, health promotion, and health services', Medical Care 23, pp. 465–583.

Kaplan R. M.: 1990, 'Behavior as a central outcome in health care', American Psychologist 45, pp. 1211–1220.

Kaplan, R. M.: 1991, 'Value for money in management of HIV: Health-related quality of life', in A. Maynard (ed.), Economic Aspects of HIV Management (Colwood Press, London).

Kaplan, R. M.: 1993, The Hippocratic Predicament: Affordability, Access, and Accountability in American Medicine (Academic Press, San Diego).

Kaplan, R. M. and J. P. Anderson: 1990, 'The general health policy model: An integrated approach', in B. Spilker (ed.), Quality of Life Assessments in Clinical Trials (Raven, New York), pp. 131–149.

Kaplan, R. M., J. P. Anderson and T. G. Ganiats: 1993, 'The quality of well-being scale: Rationale for a single quality of life index', in S. R. Walker and R. M. Rosser (eds.), Quality of Life Assessment: Key Issues in the 1990s (Kluwer Academic Publishers), pp. 65–94.

Kaplan, R. M., J. P. Anderson, A. W. Wu, W. C. Matthews, F. Kozin and D. Orenstein: 1989, 'The quality of well-being scale: Applications in AIDS, cystic fibrosis, and arthritis', Medical Care 27(3), pp. S27–S43.

Kaplan, R. M. and J. W. Bush: 1982, 'Health-related quality of life measurement for evaluation research and policy analysis', Health Psychology 1, pp. 61–80.

Kaplan, R. M., J. W. Bush and C. C. Berry: 1976, 'Health status: Types of validity for an index of well-being', Health Services Research 11, pp. 478–507.

Kaplan, R. M., J. W. Bush and C. C. Berry: 1978, 'The reliability, stability, and generalizability of a health status index', American Statistical Association, Proceedings of the Social Statistics Section, pp. 704–709.

Kaplan, R. M., J. W. Bush and C. C. Berry: 1979, 'Health status index: Category rating versus magnitude estimation for measuring levels of well-being', Medical Care 5, pp. 501–523.

Klein, R. and B. Klein: 1985, 'Vision Disorders in diabetes', in National Diabetes Data Group - Diabetes in America, NIH Publication, pp. 85–1468.

Lasker R. D.: 1993, 'The diabetes control and complications trial. Implications for policy and practice', New England Journal of Medicine 329, pp. 1035–1036.

Lewit, E. M. and D. Coate: 1982, 'The potential of using excise taxes on reducing smoking', Journal of health Economics 1, pp. 121–145.

Lipid Research Clinics Coronary Prevention Trial Results: 1984, 'I. Reduction in incidence in coronary heart disease', Journal of the American Medical Association 251, pp. 351–364.

Maynard, A.: 1991, 'Economic issues in HIV management', in A. Maynard (ed.), Economic Aspects of HIV Management (Colwood House Medical Publications, London), pp. 6–12.

McGinnis, J. M. and W. H. Foege: 1993, 'Actual causes of death in the United States', Journal of the American Medical Association 270, pp. 2207–2212.

Muldoon, M. R., S. B. Manuck and K. A. Matthews: 1990, 'Lowering cholesterol concentrations and mortality: A quantitative review of primary prevention trials', British Medical Journal 301, pp. 309–314.

National Center of Health Statistics: 1986, 'Current estimates from the national Health Interview Survey' (National Center for Health Statistics, Hyattsville, MD).

Peto, R., A. D. Lopez, J. Boreham, M. Thun and C. Heath, Jr.: 1992, 'Mortality from tobacco in developed countries: Indirect estimation from national vital statistics', Lancet 339, pp. 1268–1278.

Pierce, J. P., A. Farcas, N. Evans, C. Berry, W. Choi, B. Rosbrook, M. Johnson and D. Bal: 1992, Tobacco Use in California (California Department of Public Health, Sacramento, CA).

Richman, D. D., M. A. Fischl and M. H. Grieco et al.: 1987, 'The toxicity of azidothymidine (AZT) in the treatment of patients with AIDS and AIDS-related complex: A double-blind, placebo-controlled trial', New England Journal of Medicine 317, pp. 192–197.

Rimm, A. A.: 1985, 'Trends in cardiac surgery in the United States', New England Journal of Medicine 312, pp. 119–120.

Rokeach, M.: 1973, The Nature of Human Values (Free Press, New York).

Rosser, R.: 1993, 'The history of health related quality of life in 1-1/2 paragraphs', Journal of the Royal Society of Medicine 86, pp. 315–318.

Shade, D., J. Santiago, J. Skyler and R. Rizza: 1983, 'Effects of intensive treatment on long-term complications in intensive insulin therapy', Princeton Excerpta Medica, Chapter 5.

Schroeder S. A.: 1987, 'Strategies for reducing medical consts by changing physician's behavior', International Journal of Technology in Health Care 3, pp. 39–50.

Sick Health Services: 1988, The Economist, July 16, pp. 19–22 (anonymous).

Steering Committee of the Physicians' Health Study Research Group: 1988, 'Preliminary report: Findings from the aspirin component of the ongoing Physicians' Health Study', New england Journal of Medicine 318, pp. 262–264.

Tchobroutsky, G.: 1978, 'Relation of diabetic control to development of microvascular complications', Diabetologia 15, pp. 143–152.

Thompson, M. S., J. L. Read, H. C. Hutchings, M. Patterson and E. D. Harris, Jr.: 1988, 'The cost-effectiveness of auranofin: Results of a randomized clinical trial', Journal of Rheumatology 15, pp. 35–42.

U.S. Office on Smoking and Health: 1990, Smoking and Health, a National Status Report: A Report to congress (2nd ed.). US Department of Health and Human Services, Public Health Service, Centers for Disease Control, Center for Chronic Disease Prevention and Health Promotion, Rockville, MD.

U.S. Surgeon General: 1989, Reducing the Health Consequences of Smoking: Twenty-five Years of Progress (US Department of Health and Human Services, Centers for Disease Control, Rockville, MD).

Voulgaropolous, D., L. J. Schneiderman and R. M. Kaplan: 1989, 'Recommendations against the use of medical procedures: Evidence, judgment and ethical implications', Unpublished manuscript, University of California, San Diego.

Wallerstein, E.: 1985, 'Circumcision – The unique American medical enigma', Urological Clinics of North America 12, pp. 123–132.

Warner, K. E.: 1986, 'Smoking and health implications of a change in federal cigarette excise tax', Journal of the American Medical Association 255, pp. 1028–1032.

Wiswell, T. E. and J. D. Roscelli: 1986, 'Corroborative evidence for the decreased evidence of urinary tract infections in circumcised male infants', Pediatrics 78, pp. 96–99.

World Health Organization: 1987, Tobacco Price and the smoking Epidemic: Smoke-Free Europe (World Health Organization, Copenhagen).

World Health Organization: 1993, The HIV/AIDS Pandemic: 1993 Overview global Program on AIDS (WHO, Geneva).

Wu, A. W. et al.: 1990, 'Quality of life in a placebo-controlled trial of zidovudine in patients with AIDS and AIDS-related complex', Journal of Acquired Immune Deficiency Syndromes 3, pp. 683–690.

Division of Health Care Sciences,
Department of community and Family Medicine,
University of California,
San Diego, CA92093 - 0622,
U.S.A.

CÉLINE MERCIER

IMPROVING THE QUALITY OF LIFE OF PEOPLE
WITH SEVERE MENTAL DISORDERS

(Accepted 14 February, 1994)

ABSTRACT. In the last forty years, there has been a movement (deinstitutionalization) to displace the locus of care of people with severe and persistent mental illness from the psychiatric hospitals to more community-based networks of services. In connection with this movement, the concept of quality of life (objective and subjective) has profoundly altered the perception of the type of care that should be offered to this clientele, as well as the objectives of that care. This paper will first consider the context in which the concept of quality of life first appeared in the mental health field. The work accomplished in this area of interest over the past fifteen years will then be reviewed. Based on descriptive and comparative studies, it will be possible to identify the factors that contribute to the subjective assessment of quality of life-as-a-whole and compare quality of life in clinical and general populations and in different life settings. The paper reports what can be learned from evaluative studies about the contribution of services to quality of life, and concludes with a discussion of ways to improve the quality of life of people with severe mental disorders.

INTRODUCTION

The severely mentally ill are individuals who suffer from severe and persistent mental illness. Severity is generally determined by diagnosis (schizophrenic disorders, major affective disorders and severe person-ality disorders), disability (difficulties in fulfilling social and vocational roles), and duration of the illness (persistence of symptoms, length and number of hospitalizations). According to epidemiological studies, severely mentally ill individuals represent at least one percent of the total population.

In the last forty years, there has been a movement (deinstitutional-ization) to displace the locus of care of these people from the psychiatric

Social Indicators Research **33:** 165–192, 1994.
© 1994 *Kluwer Academic Publishers. Printed in the Netherlands.*

hospitals to more community-based networks of services. In connection with this movement, the concept of quality of life has profoundly altered the perception of the type of care that should be offered to this clientele, as well as the objectives of that care. The emergence of this issue has caused a double shift: first, from the clinical condition (pathology) to living conditions (material, physical, social and emotional well-being) and, second, from an objective assessment of services and care needs to the consumer's subjective perceptions of his or her needs. In other words, the concept of quality of life has introduced a new set of concerns about the daily life of psychiatric patients, their life experience in the community, and their perceptions of that experience.

In this paper, we will first consider the context in which the quality of life concept first appeared in the mental health field. The work accomplished in this new area of interest over the past fifteen years will then be reviewed. Based on descriptive and comparative studies, it will be possible to identify the factors that contribute to the subjective assessment of the quality of life-as-a-whole, compare quality of life in clinical and general populations, and study how different life settings can influence objective and subjective quality of life. The second, third and fourth sections of this paper will deal with those topics. The fifth section will report on what can be learned from evaluative studies about the contribution of services to the objective and subjective quality of life. The last section will discuss and suggest ways to improve the quality of life of people with severe mental disorders based on existing data.

THE EMERGENCE OF THE CONCEPT

The emergence of the concept of quality of life in relation to support and rehabilitation services is connected with the deinstitutionalization movement and, more specifically, with its consequences. The original purpose of the movement was to humanize the care given to long-term psychiatric patients by providing them with services based in the community rather than in asylum institutions. As psychiatric hospitals were gradually closed down, Community Mental Health Centers (CMHC) were to be set up, followed by Community Support Systems (CSS), to assure the social reintegration of former psychiatric patients (NIMH, 1977, 1981).

However, since these services affected only a segment of the dein-stitutionalized population, the living conditions in the communities of numerous ex-psychiatric patients were soon being described as a "national disgrace" (Reich, 1973; Talbott, 1979) and a "major social tragedy" (Lamb, 1984). These revelations led to the proposal that, in the context of deinstitutionalization (the main purpose of which was to humanize the care of long-term psychiatric patients), the evaluation of the patients' relative comfort in their non-institutional environments was equally as important as the evaluation of their clinical and functional development (Lamb, 1981).

Baker and Intagliata (1982) cited five reasons for the rapid adoption of the notion of the quality of life in the field of community psychi-atry. First, given the current state of medical knowledge, increasing the comfort of patients with severe mental disorders is a more realistic goal than "curing" them. Second, the community support programs set up to take over from the psychiatric hospitals work with a complex set of interventions. A multidimensional variable such as quality of life offers the possibility of evaluating the interaction of elements that, viewed individually, would have effects too small to perceive. Third, the concept of quality of life takes into account a new priority in pro-gram planning: client satisfaction. Forth, quality of life offers a new viewpoint that takes into account the client's life as a whole rather than concentrating solely on his or her pathology, which is in line with the holistic health perspective promoted by the World Health Organization. Lastly, talking about quality of life echoes a dominant theme in current political discourse.

The above conditions have led quality of life research to concentrate primarily on clienteles with severe, persistent mental health problems (Bachrach, 1982; Bachrach and Lamb, 1982; Mercier, 1988; Schul-berg, 1979; Schulberg and Bromet, 1981; Tantam, 1988; Wolfe and Schulberg, 1982). The descriptive, comparative and evaluate studies have focused mainly on objective and subjective living conditions in various "life domains" with respect to support services aimed at social reintegration.

More recently, the notion of subjective quality of life has also surfaced in the field of pharmacotherapy. Diamond (1985) highlighted the importance of taking the chronic psychiatric patient's point of view into account when prescribing medication. His article is a plea for the broadening of the usual criteria for medication effectiveness (the reduction of symptoms and a decrease in rehospitalization) and safety, in order to be better able to take the patient's point of view into consideration. Patients do not necessarily apply the same criteria as psychiatrists when evaluating medication: they are extremely concerned with how taking or not taking their medication will affect their quality of life. A patient may make his or her own assessment of the medication's impact on his or her life based on personal values, aspirations, current situation, and experience with other treatments, all of which will influence his or her attitudes toward pharmacotherapy (Donovan and Blake, 1992; Kaljee and Beardsley, 1992). It is important, then, to pay attention to this cost-benefit assessment, to expectations surrounding the effects of medication, and to perceptions of an acceptable level of risk and inconvenience, which can provide us with insight into the patient's compliance or resistance (Lambert, 1992; Mercier, 1989a). To date, few studies have been done on this subject, and the use of subjective quality of life criteria in clinical trials is still rare in the mental health field (Award, 1992; Gérin et al., 1992; Lepkifer et al., 1988; Meltzer et al., 1990).

THE DETERMINANTS OF QUALITY OF LIFE

One of the first descriptive studies of the quality of life of psychiatric patients was Lehman's work (Lehman et al., 1982a) with 278 residents of several board-and-care homes in Los Angeles (group homes with a minimum of 40 residents). To carry out this study, the author developed the "Quality of Life Interview" to extract demographic and clinical data and objective and subjective quality of life indicators from eight areas of life: living situation, family relations, social relations, leisure activities, work, finances, personal safety and access to legal aid, and health (Lehman, 1988). The author's intention was to test the Andrews and Withey's (1976) quality of life model and assess the relative contribution of socio-demographic characteristics and objective and subjective living conditions to global well-being (Lehman, 1983a).

The results of this study reveal how important subjective perceptions are to appreciation of life in general. An overall feeling of well-being was most closely associated with four subjective variables: satisfaction with personal health, leisure activities, social relations and financial situation. Among the objective indicators, those most closely connected to an overall feeling of well being were: not having been the victim of robbery or assault, making less use of health services, and having a greater number of satisfying social contracts in the residence, a job, and more privacy. Individual characteristics related to global well-being were: being married, having a higher level of education, and not using drugs. Although those three sets of variables accounted for between 48% and 58% of the total variance, the contribution of the subjective variables was far larger (25% to 35%) than that of the objective (7% to 16%) and individual (4% to 7%) variables. This study thus showed that the quality of life of chronic psychiatric patients was principally affected by social, not medical, problems. Moreover, patients' psychopathology had no bearing on the subjective perception of either their overall lives or the individual areas of study, except that of physical health (Lehman, 1983b).

In a Canadian study, Kearns *et al.* (1987) found that seven personal or objective variables were significantly related to satisfaction, which yielded the following profile of the most satisfied clients: They were older, able to identify several significant relationships in their lives, did not live in a lodging home, showed a certain degree of residential stability, were not on welfare, and declared that they had sufficient leisure activities.

A series of studies was conducted in Montreal with different groups of severely mentally ill patients (Mercier *et al.*, 1990).[1] Domains of everyday life were investigated in semi-structured interviews: housing, daily living (chores, food, clothing, errands, transportation), finances, health, main activity (job/school/other), use of spare time, interpersonal relationships, involvement with the judicial system, and personal safety. For each domain, multiple-response or open-ended questions were used to collect data on objective conditions, sources of satisfaction, problems, and aspirations. The interview concluded with open-ended questions about recent sources of pleasure and displeasure, aspirations, major preoccupations, projects, and perceptions of past and future life.

The interview protocol used three scales to assess quality of life: Satisfaction with Life Domains Scale (Baker and Intagliata, 1982), functional level (GAS, Endicott *et al.*, 1976), and perceived level of difficulty with daily living activities (Tessler and Goldman, 1982). A checklist helped to describe service use during the year preceding the interview. A total of 244 severely mentally ill people were involved in these studies, of whom 93 were living in Montreal, 59 in a suburb, and 92 in a remote area.

In these studies, the subjective indicators most closely related to the perception of overall quality of life were satisfaction with health, close social relationships, daily activities, and perceived level of difficulty in accomplishing daily activities. The objective indicators were functional level, age at first hospitalization, having someone to ask for small favors, and having a primary occupation (not necessarily a job). When the same data was submitted to a causal modeling analysis, the latent variable "Autonomy," namely, not living in group home, global functioning, having sufficient money and having at least one leisure activity, showed the strongest correlation (0.31) with satisfaction with life-as-a-whole (Mercier and King, 1994).

In conclusion, the areas that seem to carry the greatest weight as regards appreciation of life in general are satisfaction with health, occupation (work or principal occupation and leisure), social relations, and finances. The objective indicators cover financial situation, employment status, health, and frequency of interpersonal relationships. These indicators, however, have much less influence on the assessment of quality of life than do subjective perceptions.[2]

All life areas have not received equal attention from researchers, however. A survey of twenty descriptive studies[3] on the quality of life of severely mentally ill people living in the community (Mercier and Corten, in press), reveals that some areas are discussed in virtually every study, while others are rarely examined. Areas most frequently investigated (in 50% of studies or more) are place of residence, health, leisure and social activities, interpersonal and family relations, and finances – all domains that are directly addressed by specialized services. With regard to mental illness itself, it may seem surprising that so little interest has been shown in the patients' perceptions of their own symptoms, medication, and treatment. The clinical experience, as well as some survey data, pinpoint two areas to which more attention should undoubtedly be paid: inner or spiritual life seen as a positive value, and personal safety as a source of concern.

Another issue that needs to be addressed is the extent to which a person's functional level acts as an underlying variable affecting both objective and subjective quality of life. Certain studies show that connections exist between the level of functioning and the subjective perception of quality of life. Baker and Intagliata (1982) observed a positive correlation ($r = 0.29$) between the level of functioning as assessed by the Global Assessment Scale and the general perception of quality of life. In the Montreal study, the level of functioning measured according to the same scale (GAS) showed the same strong correlation ($r = 0.34$) with satisfaction with life, as well as with the perceived level of difficulty in accomplishing daily activities ($r = 0.45$) (Mercier et al., 1990). In the Hamilton study (Kearns et al., 1987), coping was associated with satisfaction (self-assessed, $r = 0.55$; assessed by a caregiver, $r = 0.41$).

A research team in Texas (Franklin et al., 1986) studied the relationships between objective indicators of life situations (housing, living arrangements, employment, leisure activities, income, and number of friends), the degree of satisfaction with each of these indicators, and adaptation, as measured by the perceived ability to accomplish daily living activities and scores on both the Affect Balance Scale (Bradburn, 1969) and a self-esteem scale (Rosenberg, 1965). Once again, no relationship was observed between the subjective quality of life and living conditions. There was, however, a significant relationship between degree of satisfaction and adaptation scales.

In the study by Lepkifker et al. (1988) of patients being treated with lithium, a significant positive correlation was observed between life satisfaction in general and adjustment (in terms of both over-all functioning and four specific areas: work/housework, relationship with spouse, leisure activities and interpersonal relationships), as per-ceived by patients and their psychiatrists. An Austrian study (Halford *et al.*, 1991) revealed a connection between the negative symptoms of schizophrenia (social withdrawal, difficulty in fulfilling roles, poor affective response, and apathy) and a lower objective quality of life.

All of these studies lead us to believe that a connection exists between the patient's level of functioning and the objective and subjective quality of life. The empirical data follow the lines of a proposed model of sub-jective quality of life that links level of satisfaction with a good balance between personal characteristics and environment. Bubolz *et al.* (1980) proposed an operationalization of this model for the general population. The models developed by the teams of Bigelow (1982) and Franklin (1986) were more in reference to clinical populations. According to Bigelow's model, quality of life depends on both the satisfaction of personal needs by the resources available in the environment and on individual performance, or the realization of one's abilities in response to society's demands. This model focuses more on objective quality of life. The "Oregon Quality of Life Questionnaire" is a structured interview that assesses quality of life according to this model (Bigelow *et al.*, 1990, Bigelow *et al.*, 1991a).[4]

COMPARISONS WITH THE GENERAL POPULATION

According to studies that have compared mean quality of life ratings from samples of seriously mentally ill people with national samples or non-mentally ill sub-samples (Baker and Intagliata, 1982; Huxley and Warner, 1992; Lehman *et al.*, 1982a; Mercier and Corten, 1989; Mercier *et al.*, 1992; Simpson *et al.*, 1989; Sullivan *et al.*, 1991), the evaluation of life-as-a-whole is lower among the clinical samples than among the general population. On a Likert scale (1 to 7, with 7 being the most satisfied), the general American population rated their life-as-a-whole at 5.5 (Andrews and Withey, 1976). The ratings of the clinical population through different studies ranged between 4.4 and 5.3. In comparison, the ratings of other socially disadvantaged groups in the same survey were: 5.1 for people with low socio-economic status, 5.0 for single parents, and 4.8 for Afro-Americans.

Domains rated consistently negatively provide an indication of the specific needs of people with severe mental disorders living in the community. Finances, work or daily activities, leisure and social relations, and family relations are all perceived more negatively in the clinical samples than in the general population. However, there is a striking similarity between the clinical and general populations in the domain of finances, where perceptions are the lowest for all groups (4.5 to 4.8 out of a possible 7). In Canada, compared to the general population, clinical populations have a slightly more positive perception of their quality of life in all domains pertaining to housing conditions. These somewhat surprising results show the absence of a direct relationship between objective and subjective living conditions, confirming previous observations. The clinical population may be satisfied with less than the general population. This is due, perhaps, to lowered expectations of living arrangements, loss of interest in that particular domain, or a personal preoccupation with severe and persistent mental health problems.

QUALITY OF LIFE AND ENVIRONMENT/LIVING SITUATION

From the data reported in the preceding section, it appears that quality of life ratings can be sensitive to the specific subjective experience of severely mentally ill people living in the community. Some differences can also be observed between urban and rural sub-groups of people with severe mental disorders. According to studies done in northwestern Quebec (Mercier et al., 1992) and Mississippi (Sullivan et al., 1991), rural groups have more positive perceptions of residence, neighborhood, services, clothing, health, and spare time than do urban groups. Their level of satisfaction with life in general is higher than that of the urban sample population (5.4 and 5.3 vs 4.9 and 4.4), and only marginally lower than that of the general population (5.5).

These results are in line with the few studies that have compared the living conditions of psychiatric patients in urban and rural settings to conclude that patients living in rural areas or small towns are better off than are those living in large cities. Chu *et al.* (1986) followed 275 discharged patients suffering from schizophrenia who returned to rural or urban living environments. Patients living in urban settings were perceived by their next-of-kin as being more impoverished, distressed, nervous, strange, and hyperactive compared to patients discharged to rural settings. They were also perceived as being less emotionally stable and less active in social and leisure activities. These results were confirmed by Davies *et al.* (1989), whose study showed that, compared to their rural counterparts, individuals who had received a diagnosis of schizophrenia and were living in urban settings were more likely to be living in unhealthy lodgings, receiving less help from the person in charge of the lodging, feeling different from the other residents more often, and living in less desirable neighborhoods.

A great deal can also be learned from studies that compare objective and subjective quality of life according to various types of living arrangements. Some of these studies have compared inpatient and outpatient facilities: a state psychiatric hospital and supervised community residences (Lehman *et al.*, 1986; Lehman *et al.*, 1991); acute wards in a district general hospital, a ten-bed hospital/hostel ward, and group homes (Simpson *et al.*, 1989); and patients in intensive in-house treatment, intensive outpatient treatment, and regular outpatient treatment (Warner and Huxley, 1993). Other studies were concerned with different types of living arrangements in the community: Levitt *et al.* (1990) compared sub-groups of individuals living independently, with family, and in boarding homes; the Mercier study (1989b) looked at the lives of people living alone, with their natural families (mother, father, siblings, etc.), with matrimonial families (spouse, children), or in foster homes.

Even though the above studies were carried out in three different countries (England, Canada and the United States), their conclusions are surprisingly similar: the hospitalized patients' perception of their quality of life was more negative than that of patients living in the community (Lehman *et al.*, 1986, 1991; Simpson *et al.*, 1989). Among non-hospitalized patients, those living in more structured environments, such as hostel-wards (Simpson *et al.*, 1989), intensive in-house treatment centers (Warner and Huxley, 1993), and boarding homes (Levitt *et al.*, 1990; Mercier, 1989b), were less satisfied than those living in less restricted environments.

Two of the studies (Mercier and Simpson) are more explicit about objective conditions in different types of living arrangements, clarifying the advantages and constraints of different milieus. For example, Simpson's study found that although people living in group homes had more social contacts, they also had to contend with less cohesion and more intrusion, while patients in hostel/ward units had access to more leisure activities than did others and were less likely to be victims of robbery. People living in group homes and hostel/psychiatric units also lived in greater comfort than hospitalized psychiatric patients.

In our Montreal study, the 152 participants (suffering from schizophrenia and bipolar disorders) belonged to one of four groups: those living alone (18.9%), with their natural families (parental homes: mother, father, siblings, etc.) (11.2%), with a spouse or child(ren) (matrimonial homes) (32.5%), and in foster homes (38.4%).

When the groups were compared between each other and with a sample of homeless individuals (Fournier, 1989), findings indicated that subjects' living arrangements contributed to the definition of their lifestyle and their particular mode of social reintegration. Of the four groups, the one living in matrimonial homes expressed the highest level of satisfaction. Participants belonging to this group were the most functional and had the lowest rate of hospitalization. Their residential stability was the highest of all the groups, they visited friends more often, and were involved in a variety of activities. They owned or had access to many consumer goods, such as electronic equipment, cars, bicycles, pets, plants, and home and life insurance. It seems reasonable to say that respondents living in matrimonial homes most closely resembled the general population both clinically and functionally, as well as with regard to material living conditions and social life.

The least satisfied participants in many domains were those who lived in parental homes, even though their material living conditions and residential stability were similar to those of participants living in matrimonial homes. Although they knew their neighbors, they shared few activities with them. More than half of this group had no leisure activities (53.5%).

Participants living in foster homes experienced more hospitalizations and had low residential stability and few material resources. The proportion of respondents in this group who said they did not have enough to live on was higher: 31.9% as opposed to 26.9% of those living alone, 20.0% of those living with their natural family and 8.7% of those living in a matrimonial family. The foster home group had a very small proportion (6.5%) with access to a car, as compared to 61.7% of people living in matrimonial families, and the lowest proportion of individuals with some sort of leisure activities (35.4%) or social interactions (visits, phone calls, parties). In spite of these figures, however, they were more satisfied with their living conditions than were respondents in parental homes.

The situation of those living alone seems rather precarious with respect to housing and material living conditions. For some people, this instability appears to be compensated for by participation in leisure activities and increased neighborhood involvement. This group is the one most involved in sports (46.2%), hobbies (46.2%), leisure centers (30.8%), and clubs (34.6%). The higher level of social interaction may compensate for a lack of material goods; people living alone are obliged to rely on others for such amenities as the use of a telephone or a lift to the grocery store. It goes without saying that this type of living arrangement can stimulate social reintegration only in accepting environments.

All these observations illustrate the heterogeneity of the population in need of services. If we look at the studies more closely, it appears that people living in the most structured environments are the least satisfied with their living conditions and afflicted with the most severe problems. The vast majority of the hospitalized patients in Lehman's and Simpson's studies were individuals suffering from schizophrenia, scoring lowest on the Global Assessment Scale (GAS, Endicott *et al.*, 1976). Similarly, in the Mercier study, individuals living with their parents or in foster homes had the most severe psychiatric antecedents and were the least functional, while those living with a spouse and child(ren) had the fewest disabilities. These findings appear to confirm the consistently observed relationship between functional level and subjective quality of life.

The fact that the parental home environment is richer in resources than foster homes did not positively affect respondents' perceptions. By contrast, those living in foster homes seem to have learned to be content with little. These paradoxical results could perhaps be explained by differences in subjects' aspirations and expectations.

The studies all stress that the use of services plays a significant role in the client's general living context. One service can respond to many different needs, depending on the living conditions of its recipients. For a person living in a foster home, for example, participation in activities at a day center can fulfil his or her need for stimulation, while for those living in parental homes, the center provides a change of scene. Individuals living alone can appreciate other aspects of the center, such as community meals, leisure activities, and training in social skills – all of which would help compensate for their precarious living conditions. For those living in matrimonial homes, the day center could serve as a transitional environment following hospitalization. In all cases, the relevance of any given service is measured by its versatility.

THE CONTRIBUTIONS OF SERVICES TO QUALITY OF LIFE

One of the first evaluative studies to look at the impact of services on quality of life was Stein and Test's research on the Training in Community Living program (1980). Their study dealt with such objective variables as place of residence, leisure activities, quality of milieu and employment, as well as one subjective variable: life satisfaction. Although some subsequent studies have also examined the impact of services on objective living conditions (Bigelow and Young, 1991; Bigelow et al., 1991b; Franklin, Solovitz et al., 1987; Goering et al., 1988), most studies have used both objective and subjective indicators. The specialized literature contains more than 25 articles that present evaluation results based on quality of life criteria.[5]

In general, the literature shows that programs of community support services or case management are effective in improving the quality of life of chronic psychiatric patients. An analysis of the type of variables that present consistently positive results can help identify areas where the needs of chronic psychiatric patients can be met (or, at least, partially fulfilled) by mental health services. On the other hand, variables that consistently present mixed, non-significant or negative results call attention to needs on which existing services have less impact.

Areas where positive impact is most evident are interpersonal relations (12 positive, 10 non-significant), psychological well-being (18 positive, 11 non-significant), and hobbies (5 positive, 1 non-significant). Results are more ambiguous in the areas of employment and education (5 positive and 10 non-significant), satisfaction of basic needs (3 positive, 2 negative, 6 non-significant), household maintenance (3 positive, 5 non-significant), and finances (4 positive, 8 non-significant). These last areas fall outside the specific area of health services; they are affected by policies governing income security, job accessibility, education, and housing. It is possible that these more general political and economic factors have a negative effect on the overall impact of specialized services on specific target populations.

Internal subjective processes could also contribute to negative assessments. Domains where services represent exceptional measures (as compared to the general population) give recipients the impression of living in the community, but always "on the fringe" – outside of the mainstream. The resulting subjective perception of the quality of life in the corresponding domain thus tends to be negative. For instance, some users of vocational programs have few illusions regarding their activities in sheltered workshops, jokingly referring to them as "Mickey Mouse jobs."

In fact, it is not at all certain that a direct relationship exists between participation in a service and an improved subjective quality of life in the corresponding life domain. Studies in Montreal and the United States have shown that there is no direct link between receiving services in a given life area and the perception of quality of life in that same area (Bigelow and Young, 1991; Bigelow et al., 1991b; Bond et al., 1988; Cutler et al., 1987; Field and Yegge, 1982; Franklin et al., 1987; Huxley and Warner, 1992). In the Montreal study, it was surprising to note that the more participants used rehabilitation services, the less satisfied they were with their quality of life in the areas of daily occupations and activities, free time, and life in general. On the whole, the more individuals made use of services, the more negative their perception of their quality of life became. This statement could also be reversed to suggest that a positive perception of quality of life in various areas leads to less use of services in exactly those areas (Hachey and Mercier, 1993).

These remarks are not meant to imply that we should focus less on users' actual living conditions. On the contrary, the improvement of objective living conditions should remain a service objective. We cannot expect, however, that an improvement in patients' living conditions will necessarily result in their greater satisfaction. The concepts of personal aspirations and subjective importance are particularly helpful in understanding why there is not a more direct relation between intervention and a change in how a patient perceives his or her quality of life, or between objective living conditions and subjective quality of life.

According to authors interested in subjective quality of life among the general population (Campbell *et al.*, 1976; Emmons *et al.*, 1985; Michalos, 1980, 1985), individuals' assessment of their quality of life (in general or in specific areas) is a function of perceived discrepancies between their actual lives (current situation) and what they think their lives should be (personal aspirations). These aspirations can be based on better situations in the past, the situations of friends and family, the average situation in the individual's milieu, or what he or she expects for the future. It also appears that human beings adapt to events, readjusting their aspirations and expectations to external conditions or personal realities. Thus, a person who becomes disabled because of an accident will lower his or her expectations correspondingly and, consequently, be satisfied with less. Inversely, lottery winners will invariably raise their expectations to match their new financial status (Brickman *et al.*, 1978). Calman (1984) has shown that, in the case of cancer patients, the gap between expectations and accomplishments can vary depending on whether their health is improving or deteriorating as a result of treatment or progress of the disease.

These results show that people who say they are satisfied with their quality of life in spite of adverse objective situations may have lowered their expectations following a process of learned helplessness. In the case of such individuals, rehabilitation could consist in inspiring a higher level of expectations, which would inevitably result in a certain degree of dissatisfaction over the short term. In any circumstance, it seems important to question not only the relevance of a service (its ability to meet needs), but also its significance for the recipient (its ability to fulfil aspirations and expectations).

There is one area where the contribution of services to the quality of life has been greatly neglected: mental health services. According to an American study, more than half of the daily events reported by psychiatric outpatients were related to the use of a service (Baker *et al.*, 1985). Services are therefore more than a means to a better quality of life; they are direct participants in that quality of life, a finding confirmed in the Montreal study.

The participants in this study were asked to identify people who were important to them in relation to certain parameters: the most important people in their lives, those to whom they talked when they had problems, those on whom they called in emergency situations, and those whom they asked for help with certain tasks. Although the family of origin still holds the place of honor in the support network, professionals and friends also figure prominently when it comes to finding someone with whom to discuss personal problems. In emergency situations, professionals and para-professionals represent an important source of help, in addition to family and friends. Given the important role they play in their clients' lives, workers in mental health services are thus directly implicated in their quality of life.

IMPROVING QUALITY OF LIFE

The interest in the quality of life of people with severe, persistent mental health problems is connected to the objectives of social reintegration. The interest in living conditions and the focus on personal perceptions spring from the assumption that if people undergoing the process of social reintegration are satisfied with their living conditions, their positive perception will help keep them in the community.

Studies on the determinants of subjective quality of life show the importance of perceptions over socio-demographic characteristics and objective living conditions in the assessment of quality of life. They also call attention to patients' adaptation and perceived ability to carry out daily activities and fulfil roles. From this perspective, the research on quality of life can contribute significantly to the assessment of needs of people with severe mental disorders (Cheng, 1988). The use of objective and subjective indicators enhances the information value of each type of indicator, resulting in a more detailed perspective on patients' needs. Cheng (1988) proposed the combining of objective and subjective indicators along two axes: satisfactory/unsatisfactory (subjective) and adequate/deficient (objective).

The life domains with which people with severe mental disorders express strong dissatisfaction correspond to the traditional spheres of intervention: health, employment, principal occupation and leisure, social relations, and finances. Open questions about participants' general perception of life confirm the importance of these domains in their lives. The two domains that raise the most concern are health and access to employment and education. The domains that participants most strongly wish to change or improve are primarily work and material conditions. It is also in relation to these two areas, as well as those of health, personal growth and romantic interest, that people interviewed make the most plans (Mercier *et al.*, 1990).

There are certain domains, such as selfhood (Cheng, 1988), medication (Diamond, 1985), spirituality, personal safety, and defense of rights, that have received relatively little attention from either researchers or practitioners. These domains could have a significant impact (positive or negative) on the patients' quality of life. Based on Lehman's findings concerning the victimization of psychiatric patients, one-third of the participants in his study had been robbed or assaulted during the previous year (Lehman and Linn, 1984), a special case should be made for personal safety. In the Montreal survey, 61.8% of the respondents had had contact with the police in the previous year. Over half of those contacts (55.2%) had been initiated as the result of a criminal offense: creating a disturbance (33.3%), theft (28.9%), and various disdemeanors (drunkenness, vagrancy, and possession of stolen goods) (28.9%). However, the large proportion (44.8%) of contacts with the police that occurred because the patient was in the position of victim or in need of assistance attests to the vulnerability of former psychiatric patients. A significant proportion of the sample had also been attacked or robbed (17.5%), or had lent money (22.1%) or possessions (17.4%) which had never been returned. Over a quarter of the respondents (28.7%) found it very difficult to defend their rights.

More specialized studies within a specific domain (living situation, for example) can shed new light on the fit between personal characteristics, needs and resources, palliative services, and objective and perceived living conditions. For example, perception studies have shown that residence appreciation criteria have less to do with the actual facilities than with such factors as safety, privacy, and minimal restrictions.

If one considers that the evaluation of quality of life is a dynamic process based on aspirations and the relative importance assigned to certain life domains, then quality of life has something to do with quality of care. Since people with severe mental disorders have few means and very little control over their environment, they need support to develop strategies to fulfil their personal values and aspirations. Interventions aimed at improving quality of life could have the objective of optimizing patients' strategies from several different angles: taking into consideration their attitudes, personal preferences and sources of satisfaction, and the mobilizing of their expectations towards the attainment of their own goals; improving their personal behavior and usual daily living strategies; supporting them in their current and potential alliances with people in their milieu; and maintaining or enhancing the quality of life of family, friends, natural caregivers and helpers.

The quality of life model based on adaptation provides a stimulating frame of reference to actualize these objectives. As mentioned earlier, this model defines quality of life in terms of the relationship between, on the one hand, a person's needs and available resources and, on the other hand, his or her performance and expectations of his or her environment. From the perspective of this model, mental health care work encompasses much more than direct services. It includes: (1) negotiation between the patient's demands and needs and the community's resources and possibilities; (2) development of skills required to meet the expectations of the environment and take advantage of available resources; and (3) development of the resources and expectations in the psychiatric patients' environment in order to create a real place for them in society. After all, the recognition of one's individual place in one's own environment is the foundation of quality of life.

RECOMMENDATIONS

In the light of the expertise developed through studies on the quality of life of people with severe mental disorders, specific recommendations may be made. These recommendations pertain to four separate but related issues: the types of service to be developed, the components of rehabilitation programs, the centering of services on clients, and the quality of service environment.

Recommendation 1: Descriptive studies have shown us how people with severe mental disorders living in the community perceive their lives. Study participants expressed distinct dissatisfaction with certain life domains: work, leisure activities, significant social relationships, and income. These domains all correspond to types of service that should be given priority when designing programs.

Recommendation 2: In the area of rehabilitation services, every intervention aimed at improving skills and abilities should have an impact on quality of life through the enhancement of functional level. It appears, however, that the better a rehabilitation intervention corresponds to a client's areas of personal interest, the more impact it will have on his or her quality of life. Rehabilitation work would thus have much to gain from concentrating on clients' interests and personal aspirations.

Recommendation 3: When the notion of quality of life is seen as a dynamic process based on clients' personal goals and interests, it can do much to re-focus services on clients. Users' assessment of the quality of service received is based on the extent to which they are treated as human beings who have already devised personalized courses of action to fulfill their values and desires. When it comes to developing such strategies, however, people with severe mental disorders have very few means at their disposal and even less control over their environment to do so (Lecomte, 1991). An intervention centered on quality of life aimed at optimizing existing strategies would be carried out at three different levels: (1) identifying clients' hopes and aspirations in order to put them in perspective based on real possibilities and mobilize them in personal projects; (2) recognizing clients' behaviour and usual strategies for dealing with daily life in order to increase their effectiveness and multiply sources of satisfaction; and (3) acknowledging existing and potential alliances with people in clients' milieus in order to optimize adaptation strategies.

Recommendation 4: Lastly, it would be wrong to conclude that services are no more than a means to their users' improved quality of life; they are in fact active participants. Studies have shown that psychiatric patients consider service providers to be among the most important people in their support network. Special attention should therefore be paid to a service's physical, material and organizational environment and the well-being of its workers as they have a direct effect on the quality of life of its users.

CONCLUSIONS

In the field of mental health, the concept of quality of life has created new approaches to dealing with the service needs of severely mentally disordered people. In the early 1980s, many authors proposed that the notions of cure and progress had a relative pertinence for chronic mental patients, and that an important step would be accomplished towards the humanization of services if they could "only" maintain and enhance the quality of life of this clientele. Quality of life then became a major issue in the assessment of the patients' need and of the impact of services on their lives. This new approach has been reflected in recent mental health policies and program objectives.

In this paper, we addressed the historical and current use of the concept of quality of life in research on services. The value of quality of life assessments in the care and management of severely mentally disordered people has to be seen within their wider context: a background of long-stay hospital closure and the transition to community care, a heavily stigmatized client group that has difficulty attracting staff and funding, and inter-organizational gaps in service delivery that pose considerable challenges for comprehensiveness and continuity of care.

When used for planning purposes, the studies on quality of life all share an emphasis on the point of view of the clients – their preferences, aspirations, limitations, and personal projects. The concern for quality of life draws attention to the ecological dimension of services, which should fit the clients' social, cultural, and material conditions. Both objective and subjective factors can influence clients' perceptions of whether or not interventions have an impact on their quality of life.

As a final comment, we would like to propose that the next step in the issue of quality of life and the severely mentally disordered should be community-oriented. Past experience suggests that services contribute to the improvement of living conditions and to the development of competence, and that they can facilitate life in the community. The role of families, neighbors, natural helpers and lay people is also essential. In fact, only the environment in which people with severe mental disorders live has the potential to support their efforts to attain full recognition from society. Intervention strategies should also be developed to help communities become "competent communities" for their members-in-need.

ACKNOWLEDGMENTS

This work was made possible by a *Bourse d'excellence* in evaluation from the *Conseil québécois de la recherche sociale*. I also wish to thank Cynthia Gates for her editing assistance with regard to the English language.

NOTES

[1] This research was supported by grants from Conseil québécois de la recherche sociale (Quebec Health and Social Services Ministry), National Welfare Grant Program (Health and Welfare Canada) and from Collaborative Research Grant (NATO).

[2] These results are in accordance with surveys in general population where most demographic characteristics and objective life situations are not significantly related to the overall subjective quality of life. Satisfaction with marriage and family life are the best predictors of global satisfaction with life (Campbell *et al.*, 1976; Diener, 1984).

[3] The following studies have been considered: Delespaul and DeVries, 1987; Earls and Nelson, 1988; Fabian, 1989; Frankin *et al.*, 1986; Gaglione and Horassius, 1991; Gluge *et al.*, 1985; Godin-Azis *et al.*, 1992; Huxley and Warner, 1992; Lehman *et al.*, 1982 a, b; Lehman, 1983 a, b; Lehman and Linn, 1984; Lehman *et al.*, 1986; Levitt *et al.*, 1990; Mercier, 1989 b; Mercier *et al.*, 1992; Simpson *et al.*, 1989; Skantze *et al.*, 1992; Spivack *et al.*, 1982; Sullivan *et al.*, 1991; Thapa and Rowland, 1989.

[4] Heinrichs *et al.* (1984), and Malm *et al.* (1981) have also developed tools to assess objective quality of life. The psychometric properties of these instruments, as well the ones of five others (including Lehman's Quality of Life Interview and Baker and Intagliata's Satisfaction with Life Domain Scale) are described in Lehman and Burns (1990) and in Bell (1993). Oliver (1992) also developed a Quality of Life Profile for the evaluation of community services for the mentally ill. Tools available in French (translation or originals) are described in Mercier and Corten (in press).

[5] Besides the studies cited in this section, the following may be mentioned: Baker and Intagliata, 1982; Baker *et al.*, 1992; Dalgard, 1983; Dickey *et al.*, 1981; Gibbons and Butler, 1987; Mercier *et al.*, 1992; Okin *et al.*, 1983, 1993; Pinkney *et al.*, 1991; Solomon, 1992; Wright *et al.*, 1989.

REFERENCES

Andrews, F. M. and S. B. Withey: 1976, Social Indicators of Well-Being (Plenum Press, New York).

Awad, A. G.: 1992, 'Quality of life of schizophrenic patients on medications and implications for new drug trials', Hospital and Community Psychiatry 43(3), pp. 262–265.

Bachrach, L. L.: 1982, 'Assessment of outcomes in community support systems: results, problems and limitations', Schizophrenia Bulletin 8(1), pp. 39–61.

Bachrach, L. L. and H. R. Lamb: 1982, Conceptual issues in the evaluation of the deinstitutionalization movement, in G. J. Stahler and W. R. Tash (eds.), Innovation Approaches to Mental Health Evaluation (Academic Press, New York) pp. 139–161.

Baker, F. and J. Intagliata: 1982 'Quality of life in the evaluation of community support systems', Evaluation and Program Planning 5, pp. 69–79.

Baker, F., T. F. Burns, M. Libby and J. Intagliata: 1985, 'The impact of life events on chronic mental patients', Hospital and Community Psychiatry 36(3), pp. 299–301.

Baker, F., D. Jodrey and J. Intagliata: 1992, 'Social support and quality of life of community support clients', Community Mental Health Journal 28(5), pp. 397–411.

Bell, R.: 1993, 'Un aperçu des théories et des mesures de qualité de vie pour l'évaluation des services psychiatriques', Santé mentale au Québec XVII(2), pp. 87–108.

Bigelow, D. A., G. Brodsky, L. Steward and M. Olson: 1982, 'The concept and measurement of quality of life as a dependent variable in evaluation of mental health services', in G. J. Stahler and W. R. Tash (eds.), Innovative Approaches to Mental Health Evaluation (Academic Press, New York) pp. 345–366.

Bigelow, D. A., M. J. Gareau and D. J. Young: 1990, 'A quality of life interview for chronically mentally disabled people', Psychosocial Rehabilitation Journal 14(2), pp. 94–98.

Bigelow, D. A., B. H. McFarland and M. M. Olson: 1991a, 'Quality of life of community mental health program clients: Validating a measure', Community Mental Health Journal 27(1), pp. 43–55.

Bigelow, D. A., B. H. McFarland, M. J. Gareau and D. J. Young: 1991b, 'Implementation and effectiveness of a bed reduction project', Community Mental Health Journal 27(2), pp. 125–133.

Bigelow, D. A. and D. J. Young: 1991, 'Effectiveness of a case management program', Community Mental Health Journal 27(2), pp. 115–123.

Bond, G. R., L. D. Miller, M. H. A. Krumwied and R. S. Ward: 1988, 'Assertive case management in three CHMCs: A controlled study', Hospital and Community Psychiatry 39(4), pp. 411–418.

Bradburn, N. M.: 1969, The Structure of Psychological Well-Being (Aldine).

Brickman, P., D. Coates and R. Janoff-Bulman: 1978, 'Lottery winners and accident victims: Is happiness relative', Journal of Personality and Social Psychology 36, pp. 917–927.

Bubolz, M., J. Eicher, J. Evers and M. Sontag: 1980, 'A human ecological approach to quality of life: Conceptual framework and results of a preliminary study', Social Indicators Research 7, pp. 103–116.

Calman, K. C.: 1984, 'Quality of life in cancer patients. An hypothesis', Journal of Medical Ethics 10, pp. 124–127.

Campbell, A., P. E. Converse and W. L. Rogers: 1976, The Quality of American Life (Russell Sage Foundation).

Cheng, S. T.: 1988, 'Subjective quality of life in the planning and evaluation of programs', Evaluation and Program Planning 11, pp. 123–134.

Chu, C. C., H. S. Sallack and H. E. Klein: 1986, 'Differences in symptomatology and social adjustment between urban and rural schizophrenics', Social Psychiatry 21, pp. 10–14.

Cutler, D., E. Tantum and J. Shore: 1987, 'A comparison of schizophrenia patients in different community support treatment approaches', Community Mental Health Journal 23, pp. 103–113.

Dalgard, O. G.: 1983, 'Measures of psychiatric illness, mental health and quality of life', in B. Cronholm and L. V. Knorring (eds.), Evaluation of Mental Health Services Programs (Stockholm: Sweedish Medical Research Council: Proceedings from a Sweedish Medical Research Council Symposium), pp. 127–134.

Davies, M. A., E. J. Bromet, S. C. Schulz, L. O. Dunn and M. Morgenstern: 1989, 'Community adjustment of chronic schizophrenic patients in urban and rural settings', Hospital and Community Psychiatry 40(8), pp. 824–830.

Delespaul, P. A. and M. W. De Vries: 1987, 'The daily life of ambulatory chronic mental patients', Journal of Nervous and Mental Disease 175(9), pp. 537–544.

Diamond, R.: 1985, 'Drugs and the quality of life: The patient's point of view', Journal of Clinical Psychiatry 46(5), pp. 29–35.

Dickey, B., J. E. Guderman, S. Hellman, A. Donatelle and L. Grenspoon: 1981, 'A follow-up of deinstitutionalized chronic patients four years after discharge', Hospital and Community Psychiatry 32(5), pp. 326–330.

Diener, E.: 1984, 'Subjective well-being', Psychological Bulletin 95, pp. 542–575.

Donovan, J. L. and D. R. Blake: 1992, 'Patient non-compliance: Deviance or reasoned decision-making?', Social Science of Medicine 34(5), pp. 507–513.

Earls, M. and G. Nelson: 1988, 'The relationship between long-term psychiatric clients' psychological well-being and their perceptions of housing and social support', American Journal of Community Psychology 16(2), pp. 279–293.

Emmons, R. A., E. Diener and R. J. Larsen: 1985, 'Choice of situations and congruence models of interactionism', Personality and Individual Differences 6, pp. 693–702.

Endicott, J., R. L. Spitzer, J. L. Fleiss and J. Cohen: 1976, 'The global assessment scale. A procedure for measuring overall severity of psychiatric disturbance', Archives of General Psychiatry 33, pp. 766–771.

Fabrian, E. S.: 1989, 'Work and the quality of life', Psychosocial Rehabilitation Journal 12(4), pp. 39–49.

Field, G. and L. Yegge: 1982, 'A client outcome study of a community support demonstration project', Psychosocial Rehabilitation Journal VI(2), pp. 15–22.

Fournier, L.: 1989, 'La clientèle des refuges de Montréal', Thèse de doctorat en administration de la santé, Université de Montréal.

Franklin, J. L., J. Simmons, B. Solovitz, J. R. Clemons and G. E. Miller: 1986, 'Assessing quality of life of the mentally ill: A three-dimensional model', Evaluation and the Health Professions 9(3), pp. 376–388.

Franklin, J. L., B. Solovitz, M. Mason, J. R. Clemons and G. E. Miller: 1987, 'An evaluation of case management', American Journal of Public Health 77(6), pp. 674–678.

Gaglione, J. M. and M. Horassius: 1991, 'Une étude évaluative de la qualité de vie des malades mentaux chroniques', L'Information Psychiatrique 6, pp. 565–567.

Gérin, P., A. Dazord, A. Sali and J. -P. Boissel: 1992, 'L'évaluation de la dépression à la lumiére du concept de la qualité de la vie subjective', L'Information Psychiatrique 68(5), pp. XLVII–LVI.

Gibbons, J. S. and J. P. Butler: 1987, 'Quality of life for "new" long-stay psychiatric inpatients: the effects of moving to a hostel', British Journal of Psychiatry 151, pp. 347–354.

Gluge, M., V. Kovess and J. De Verbizier: 1985, 'La vie quotidienne des patients d'un hôpital de jour', Social Psychiatry 20, pp. 70–75.

Goering, P. N., D. A. Wasylenki, M. Farkas and W. J. Lancee et al.: 1988, 'Does case management make a difference?', Hospital and Community Psychiatry 39(3), pp. 272–276.

Godin-Azis, A., G. Bleirad, M. Bringau, V. Kovess, A. Mouchel and J. DeVerbizier: 1992, 'Qualité de la vie des patients d'un hôpital de jour dans la commuanuté', L'Information Psychiatrique 68(5), pp. XXVII–XXXII.

Hachey, R. and C. Mercier: 1993, 'The impact of rehabilitation services on the quality of life of chronic mental patients', Occupational Therapy in Mental Health 13(2), pp. 1–26.

Halford, W. K., R. D. Schweitzer and F. N. Varghese: 1991, 'Effects of family environment on negative symptoms and quality of life of psychotic patients', Hospital and community Psychiatry 42(12), pp. 1241–1247.

Heinrichs, D. W., T. E. Hanlon and W. T. Carpenter: 1984, 'The quality of life scale: an instrument for rating the schizophrenia deficit syndrome', Schizophrenia Bulletin 10(3), pp. 388–398.

Huxley, P. and R. Warner: 1992, 'Case management, quality of life, and satisfaction with services of long-term psychiatric patients', Hospital and Community Psychiatry 43(8), pp. 799–802.

Kaljee, L. M. and R. Beardsley: 1992, 'Psychotropic drugs and concepts of compliance in a rural mental health clinic', Medical Anthropology Quarterly 6(3), pp. 271–287.

Kearns, R. A., S. M. Taylor and M. Dear: 1987, 'Coping and satisfaction among the chronically mentally disabled', Canadian Journal of community Mental Health 6(2), pp. 13–25.

Lamb, H. R.: 1981, 'What did we really expect from deinstitutionalization?', Hospital and community Psychiatry 32(2), pp. 105–109.

Lamb, H. R.: 1984, The Homeless Mentally Ill. A Task Force of the American Psychiatric Association, American Psychiatric Association.

Lambert, A. F.: 1992, 'De quelques considérations pharmacologiques sur la qualité de la vie. A propos du valpromide', L'information psychiatrique 68(5), pp. V.

Lecomte, Y.: 1991, 'Les mécanismes d'adaptation des malades mentaux chroniques à la vie quotidienne', Santé mentale au Québec XVI(2), pp. 99–120.

Lehman, A. F., N. C. Ward and L. S. Linn: 1982a, 'Chronic mental patients: The quality of life issue', American Journal of Psychiatry 139(10), pp. 1271–1276.

Lehman, A. F., S. K. Reed and S. M. Possidente: 1982b, 'Priorities for long-term care:

Comments from board-and-care residents', Psychiatric Quarterly 54(3), pp. 181–190.

Lehman, A. F.: 1983a, 'The well-being of chronic mental patients. Assessing their quality of life', Archives of General Psychiatry 40, pp. 369–373.

Lehman, A. F.: 1983b, 'The effects of psychiatric symptoms on quality of life assessments among the chronic mentally ill', Evaluation and Program Planning 6, pp. 143–151.

Lehman, A. F. and L. S. Linn: 1984, 'Crimes against discharged mental patients in board-and-care homes', American Journal of Psychiatry 141(2), pp. 271–275.

Lehman, A. F., S. Possidente and F. Hawker: 1986, 'The quality of life of chronic patients in a state hospital and in community residences', Hospital and community Psychiatry 37(9), pp. 901–907.

Lehman, A. F.: 1988, 'A quality of life interview for the chronically mentally ill', Evaluation and Program Planning 11(1), pp. 51–62.

Lehman, A. F. and B. J. Burns: 1990, 'Severe mental illness in the community', in B. Spilker (eds.), Quality of Life Assessments in Clinical Trials (Raven Press Ltd, New York, NY), pp. 357–362.

Lehman, A. F., J. G. Slaughter and C. P. Myers: 1991, 'Quality of life in alternative residential settings', Psychiatric Quarterly 62(1), pp. 35–49.

Lepkifker, E., N. Horesh and S. Floru: 1988, 'Life satisfaction and adjustment in lithium-treated affective patients in remission', Acta Psychiatrica Scandinavica 78, pp. 391–395.

Levitt, A. J., T. P. Hogan and C. Bucosky: 1990, 'Quality of life in chronically ill patients in day treatment', Psychological Medicine 20, pp. 703–710.

Malm, N., P. R. May and S. Denaker: 1981, 'Evaluation of the quality of life of the schizophrenic out-patient: a checklist', Schizophrenia Bulletin 7(3), pp. 477–485.

Meltzer, H. Y., S. Burnett, B. Bastani and L. F. Ramirez: 1990, 'Effects of six months of clozapine treatment on the quality of life of chronic schizophrenic patients', Hospital and Community Psychiatry 41(8), pp. 892–897.

Mercier, C.: 1988, 'Le patient psychiatrique dans la communauté: son expérience de vie', L'Information psychiatrique 10, pp. 1301–1308.

Mercier, C.: 1989a, 'Le rôle des facteurs subjectifs dans la fidélité à la médication', Revue Canadienne de Psychiatrie 34(7), pp. 662–668.

Mercier, C.: 1989b, 'Conditions de vie et lieux de résidence', Santé mentale au Québec XIV(2), pp. 158–171.

Mercier, C. and P. Corten: 1989, 'Quality of life and social reintegration: Canadian and Belgian surveys with the severely mentally ill' (41st Institute on Hospital and Community Psychiatry, Philadelphia, PA).

Mercier, C. and S. King: 1994, 'A latent causal model of the quality of life of psychiatric patients', Acta Psychiatrica Scandinavia 89, pp. 72–77.

Mercier, C., Corten P.: in press, 'Évaluation de la qualité de vie de patients psychiatriques', in V. Kovess (ed.), L'Évaluation des soins en psychiatrie (Presses Universitaires de France, Paris).

Mercier, C., C. Renaud, F. Desbiens and S. Gervais: 1990, 'La contribution des services à la qualité de la vie des patients psychiatriques dans la communauté', Ottawa: Santé et Bien-être social Canada, mars. English translation: 'The contribution of Services to the Quality of Life of Psychiatric Patients in the Community', Ottawa: Health and Welfare Canada.

Mercier, C., R. Tempier and C. Renaud: 1992, 'Services communautaires et qualité de la vie: une étude d'impact en région éloignée', Canadian Journal of Psychiatry/Revue canadienne de psychiatrie 37(8), pp. 553–563.

Michalos, A. C.: 1980, 'Satisfaction and happiness', Social Indicators Research 8, pp. 385–422.

Michalos, A. C.: 1985, 'Multiple discrepancies theory (MDT)', Social Indicators Research 16(4), pp. 347–414.

National Institute of Mental Health: 1977, 'The NIMH Community Support Program: Program Description', National Institute of Mental Health.

National Institute of Mental Health: 1981, 'A Network for Caring: The Community Support Program of the National Institute of Mental Health', Proceedings of the Fifth National Conference (U.S. Department of Health and Human Services, Rockville, Md).

Okin, R. L., R. J. A. Dalmie and D. T. Pearsall: 1983, 'Patient's perspectives on community alternatives to hospitalization: A follow-up study', American Journal of Psychiatry 140(11), pp. 1460–1464.

Okin, R. L. and D. Pearsall: 1993, 'Patients' perceptions of their quality of life 11 years after discharge from a state hospital', Hospital and community Psychiatry 44(3), pp. 236–240.

Oliver, J. P. J.: 1991–92, 'The social case directive: Development of a quality of life profile for use in community services for the mentally ill', Social Work & Social Sciences Review 3(1), pp. 5–45.

Pinkney, A. A., G. J. Gerber and H. G. Lafave: 1991, 'Quality of life after psychiatric rehabilitation: the clients' perspective', Acta Psychiatrica Sandinavica 83, pp. 86–91.

Reich, R.: 1973, 'Care of the chronically mentally ill. A national disgrace', American Journal of Psychiatry 130(8), pp. 911–912.

Rosenberg, M.: 1965, Society and the Adolescent Self-image (Princeton University Press, Princeton, NJ).

Schulberg, H. C.: 1979, 'Community support programs: Program evaluation and public policy', American Journal of Psychiatry 136(11), pp. 1433–1437.

Schulberg, H. C. and E. Bromet: 1981, 'Strategies for evaluating the outcome of community services for the chronically mentally ill', American Journal of Psychiatry 138(7), pp. 930–935.

Simpson, C. J., C. E. Hyde and E. B. Faragher: 1989, 'The chronically mentally ill in community facilities. A study of quality of life', British Journal of Psychiatry 154, pp. 77–82.

Skantze, K., U. Malm, S. J. Dencker, P. R. A. May and P. Corrigan: 1992, 'Comparisons of quality of life with standard of living in schizophrenic out-patients', British Journal of Psychiatry 161, pp. 797–801.

Solomon, P.: 1992, 'The closing of a state hospital: What is the quality of patients' lives one year post-release?', Psychiatric Quarterly 63(3), pp. 279–296.

Spivack, G., J. Siegel, D. Sklaver, L. Deuschle and L. Garrett: 1982, 'The long-term patient in the community: Life style patterns and treatment implications', Hospital and Community Psychiatry 33(4), pp. 291–295.

Stein, L. I. and M. A. Test: 1980, 'Alternative to mental hospital treatment: 1. conceptual model, treatment program, and clinical evaluation', Archives of General Psychiatry 37, pp. 392–397.

Sullivan, G., K. B. Wells and B. Leake: 1991, 'Quality of life of seriously mentally ill persons in Mississippi', Hospital and Community Psychiatry 42(7), pp. 752–755.

Talbott, J. A.: 1979, 'Care of the chronically mentally ill. Still a national disgrace', American Journal of Psychiatry 136(5), pp. 688–689.

Tantam, D.: 1988, 'Quality of life and the chronically mentally ill', The International Journal of Social Psychiatry 34(4), pp. 243–247.

Tessler, R. C. and H. H. Goldman: 1982, The Chronically Mentally Ill: Assessing Community Support Programs (Ballinger Publishing Company, Cambridge MA).

Thapa, K. and L. A. Rowland: 1989, 'Quality of life perspectives in long-term care: staff and patient perceptions', Acta Psychiatrica Scandinavica 80(3), pp. 267–271.

Warner, R. and P. Huxley: 1993, 'Psychopathologie et qualité de la vie chez des malades mentaux chroniques: une comparaison entre un échantillon britannique et américain', Santé mentale au Québec XVIII(2), pp. 75–86.

Wolfe, J. C. and H. C. Schulberg: 1982, 'The design and evaluation of future mental health systems', in G. J. Stahler and W. R. Tash (eds.), Innovative Approaches to Mental Health Evaluation (pp. 3–22).

Wright, G. R., J. R. Heiman, J. Shupe and G. Olvera: 1989, 'Defining and measuring stabilization of patients during 4 years of intensive community support', American Journal of Psychiatry 146(10), pp. 1293–1298.

Douglas Hospital Research Centre,
Psychosocial Research Unit,
Verdun, Quebec,
Canada H4H 1R3

ANDREW S. HALPERN

QUALITY OF LIFE FOR STUDENTS WITH DISABILITIES
IN TRANSITION FROM SCHOOL TO ADULTHOOD

(Accepted 14 February, 1994)

ABSTRACT. This paper examines quality-of-life concerns that pertain to secondary level students with disabilities who participate in high school programs in the United States. More specifically, we examine issues and programs that pertain to the "transition period" during which students leave school and begin to assume adult roles in their communities. The paper begins with an overview of major programs that have addressed this area over the past 25 years. We then present some contrasting definitions of quality of life, in order to provide a theoretical context for examining issues and concerns, ending with our recommendations for a taxonomy that can be used for operationally defining quality of life. Research findings from this perspective are presented next, followed by a discussion of ways in which quality-of-life information can be *used* to influence program and policy and policy decisions at both personal and institutional levels of discourse. We cite and describe several examples of such usage from our own experiences. The paper closes with some recommendations concerning what we must do in the future to improve quality of life for this population.

The transition from adolescence into adulthood can be a difficult time for any young person, with or without a disability. Many changes are occurring during this time of life, not the least of which is the change from attending high school to some other primary activity as a young adult. The possibilities are many, including tertiary education, entry-level job, time-out for recreation, or unfortunately for some, less adaptive endeavors such as a period of "unengagement" or, even worse, a period of self-abusive or anti-social behavior that can result in such unhappy consequences as drug abuse, criminal behaviors and eventual incarceration.

Even at its best, this period of transition is usually accompanied by a strong sense of floundering as young people attempt to sort out the

Social Indicators Research **33**: 193–236, 1994.
© 1994 *Kluwer Academic Publishers. Printed in the Netherlands.*

lessons of their childhood and move into effective adult roles in their communities. There are many influences that affect this transition, for better or for worse, including family background, quality and impact of the high school program, nature and quality of transition services that are provided, opportunities in the community that are actually available for the young person, and the readiness and motivation exhibited by the young person to move forward with his or her life.

The general purpose of this paper is to examine quality-of-life models that have guided special education and rehabilitation programs for "transitioning" adolescents and young adults in the United States during the past 30 years. Four broad topics will be explored:

* descriptions of the major school-based programs, including the ways in which they have grappled with quality-of-life issues;
* theoretical issues concerning the definition and conceptualization of quality of life;
* the use of follow-along research strategies to examine quality-of-life outcomes; and
* strategies for improving the quality of life for special education students who are in transition.

Whenever possible and appropriate, research activities directed by the author and his colleagues over the past 25 years will be incorporated into the presentation, to illustrate the points and arguments that are being developed.

MAJOR PROGRAMS ADDRESSING TRANSITION

The word "transition," as it applies to special education and rehabilitation programs, has developed 2 distinctive meanings within the United States literature. In its generic sense, transition refers to that period of time during which students leave school and begin to assume adult roles in their communities. In recent years, however, the term has also been adopted as a label for a specific program of federal support that was designed to enhance transition programs and services for adolescents and young adults with disabilities. The federal program began in 1984 (Will, 1984; Halpern, 1985). There were several important antecedent programs, however, which began during the 1960's and laid the foundation for our current efforts. The most important of these antecedent programs were called "work-study" and "career education" programs. These programs will be reviewed briefly here in order to provide a context for raising some quality-of-life issues. A more complete description can be found elsewhere (Halpern, 1992).

Work-study programs. The work-study programs emerged in the United states during the 1960's, and were designed to create an integrated academic, social and vocational curriculum, accompanied by appropriate work experience, to prepare students with mild mental retardation for eventual community adjustment. The administration of these programs was generally structured by *formal* cooperative agreements between the schools and the state rehabilitation agency (Halpern, 1973; 1974; Kolstoe and Frey, 1965). The work-study approach emerged at a time when most high school programs for students with mental retardation focused their curriculum on remedial academics and ignored such practical areas as vocational skills and independent living skills.

The goal of these programs, as mentioned above, was "community adjustment." Although never defined precisely and consensually, the term "community adjustment" was meant to include a number of "quality-of-life" domains, including employment, independent living, and personal/social adjustment. The major focus of the work-study program, however, was clearly on employment, since this is the primary outcome goal of the vocational rehabilitation agency which served as a collaborator with the schools in the implementation of the program.

Although the work-study approach was fairly successful, it died for a number of administrative reasons during the early 1970's (Halpern, 1992). The problems being addressed by this program, however, were still very much alive, and a new "career education" program was born to take up the gauntlet.

Career education programs. Unlike the work-study programs which emerged out of a grass roots collaboration between schools and rehabilitation agencies, the career education movement was born out of federal legislation. In 1977, the United States Congress passed a bill known as "the Career Education Implementation Incentive Act (Public Law 95–207)." The general purpose of this act was to focus attention on the post-school needs of *all* students, with and without disabilities. The activities and financial support stipulated through the act were limited to 5 years, after which it was hoped that state agencies and local communities would continue whatever had been started through the federal initiative (Brolin, 1983; Cegelka, 1979; Hoyt, 1982).

It is interesting to observe that a commonly accepted definition of "career education" never did emerge, in spite of substantial activity in this area during the 1970's. The definitions that emerged from the field ranged from a narrow focusing of goals on the preparation of students for paid employment to a much broader concern with all aspects of adult life. Attempting, perhaps, to mediate between these two positions, the policy adopted by the Council on Exceptional Children contains elements of both extremes:

Career education is the totality of experiences through which one learns to live a meaningful, satisfying work life. Within the career education framework, work is conceptualized as conscious effort aimed at producing benefits for oneself and for others. Career education provides the opportunity for children to learn, in the least restrictive environment possible, the academic, daily living, personal-social and occupational knowledge and specific vocational work skills necessary for attaining their highest levels of economic, personal and social fulfillment. The individual can obtain this fulfillment through work (both paid and unpaid) and in a variety of other societal roles and personal life styles including his/her pursuits as a student, citizen, volunteer, family member, and participant in meaningful leisure time activities. (Position Paper, 1978)

Before the issue of defining outcome goals would come even close to resolution, the career education movement abruptly ended in 1982, as preplanned by the federal legislation.

Transition programs. Only two years after the repeal of the Career Education Implementation Incentive Act in 1982, a new federal transition initiative emerged on the scene (Will, 1984) in the form of a "position paper" from the United States Office of Special Education and Rehabilitative Services (OSERS). This program, like its predecessors, was and still is concerned about the interface between school and the early years of adult life for young people with disabilities. The outcome originally proposed as the focus of transition services was employment. Perhaps anticipating some concern about the narrowness of this goal, the choice of employment is justified in words such as the following (Will, 1984):

This concern with employment does not indicate a lack of interest in other aspects of adult living. Success in social, personal, leisure, and other adult roles enhances opportunities both to obtain employment and enjoy its benefits ... (p. 1)

The focus on employment as a central outcome of effective transition provides an objective measure of transition success. (p. 2)

What the author of this policy seemed to be suggesting was that the non-vocational dimensions of adult adjustment are significant and important only in so far as they contribute to the ultimate goal of employment.

Comparison of the 3 movements. There are many different frames of reference that might be used to compare these 3 movements. For the purposes of this paper, however, it is most relevant to compare the manner in which the desired outcomes of the programs were conceptualized. The transition movement's early focus on employment was narrower than the stipulated goals of either the work/study or career education movements. All three movements were aware that the dimensions of adult adjustment extend beyond employment, but only the transition movement adopted a clearly restrictive position on this issue. The reason for this restrictive position was not a lack of appreciation for the complexity of adult adjustment. Rather, it was the sense of the policy makers that a more limited objective would be more feasible, fundable, and easier to evaluate than a program with multiple objectives.

As we move into the 1990's, the transition movement remains the most powerful political and programmatic force in the United States that is concerned about the interface between school and adult life for young people with disabilities. The parameters of this movement, however, have been broadened. The most recent law addressing transition was passed in 1990 and is called the "Individuals with Disabilities Education Act" (Public Law 101–476). This law extends the concept of transition in the following manner.

Transition services means a coordinated set of activities for a student, designed within an outcome oriented process, which promotes movement from school to post-school activities, including post-secondary education, vocational training, integrated employment (including supported employment) continuing and adult education, adult services, independent living or community participation. The coordinated set of activities *must*: (a) be based upon the individual student's needs; (b) take into account the student's preferences and interests; (c) *must* include instruction, community experiences, the development of employment and other post-school adult living objectives, and if appropriate, the acquisition of daily living skills and functional vocational evaluation (Section 300.18).

Although the federal legislation is obviously still quite concerned with employment as an outcome of the transition process, the language is clearly framed in a broader way to acknowledge the relevance and importance of other needs and other outcomes. Although the term "quality-of-life" is not used explicitly in the legislation, the multi-dimensional expression and validity of life goals are clearly implied. Funding opportunities that have already emerged from this legislation also make it abundantly clear that transition outcomes are now being viewed as much broader than employment.

Quality of Life

The basic intent of the programs just reviewed has always been to enhance the quality of life of adolescents and young adults and disabilities. The basic assumption, of course, is that intervention programs, such as special education and rehabilitation, are capable of influencing quality of life. The basic problem, as we have seen, is the lack of consensus over the years on what we mean by the phrase "quality of life." Various approaches have been followed, including a narrow focus on employment and a broader focus that also includes such domains as independent living and personal/social networks.

Variations in definition. When one looks at the literature on quality of life that has emerged strongly during the past few years within the field of disability, it soon becomes evident that the issues are much broader and more complex than is reflected in simply questioning the adequacy of employment as an indicator. Consider the following definitions of quality of life that have been offered:

Quality of life is a matter of subjective experience. That is to say, the concept has no meaning apart from what a person feels and experiences. As a corollary to the first proposition, people may experience the same circumstances differently. What enhances one person's quality of life may detract from another's (Taylor and Bogdan, 1990, pp. 34–35).

Quality of life can be viewed as the discrepancy between a person's achieved and their unmet needs and desires ... Quality of life can also be viewed as the degree to which an individual has control over his or her environment (Brown et al., 1988, pp. 111–112).

Quality of life represents the degree to which an individual has met his/her needs to create their own meanings so that they can establish and sustain a viable self in the social world (Parmenter, 1988, p. 9).

When an individual, with or without disabilities, is able to meet important needs in major life settings (work, school, home, community) while also satisfying the normative expectations that others hold for him or her in those settings, he or she is more likely to experience a high quality of life (Goode, 1990, p. 46).

When one examines these and other definitions for similarities and differences, a central issue quickly becomes evident. This issue can be phrased in several ways, one of which being the discrepancy between "subjective" and "objective" criteria for defining and describing quality of life. Using this frame of reference, the term "subjective" refers to the individual's point of view and the term "objective" refers to a societal point of view. The difference is illustrated well by a model that was proposed by MacFarlane et al. (1989) and is presented below in Figure 1. Similar distinctions can be found in models that have been developed by Parmenter (1988), Goode (1990) and Schalock (1990).

As the model in Figure 1 clearly indicates, the subjective dimensions can only be ascertained from a person's own point of view, whereas the objective dimensions are accessible either from a personal perspective or someone else's perspective. The issue that has emerged is reflected in the definition presented above by Taylor and Bogdan (1990). In essence, they assert that *only* a personal perspective is relevant. This

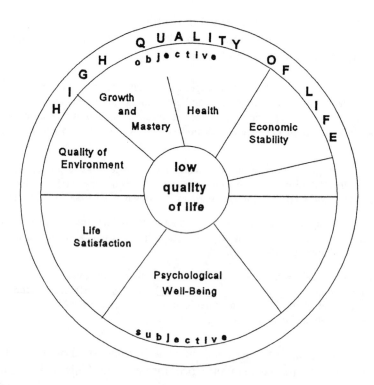

Fig. 1. Conceptual model illustrating subjective and objective dimensions of quality of life.

same approach is illustrated well in an anecdote provided by Edgerton (1990) about a 58 year old man with an IQ of 54.

He lives in a single room occupancy hotel in a rundown and crime-ridden part of downtown Los Angeles. He has a dangerous yet personally rewarding job as the night manager of a laundromat frequented by homeless people, prostitutes, and drug dealers. His sexual partners are drug-using prostitutes, one of whom recently contracted AIDS. There is no doubt that this man works very hard for the money he makes, that he is frequently in physical danger, and that his repeated exposure to AIDS could be life threatening. Yet he lives in a network of friends and acquaintances who value his friendship and help, and who do not know or care that he can neither read nor write. To many people, he is loved and respected. He is as satisfied with the quality of his life as anyone I know (p. 151).

Edgerton's point, obviously, is that this man would be viewed as experiencing a very low quality of life, if the criteria used for evaluation included such categories as *safety* and *healthy intimate relationships*. Another way of considering this underlying issue is to examine the role of personal *choice* in determining the quality of life.

At one level of analysis, personal choice is presumed by any quality-of-life model that includes subjective perspectives as part or all of the underlying definition. The major point of Edgerton's anecdote was to illustrate the tension between an individual's choices and societal norms. Edgar (1987) illustrates the same tension when he explores some possible consequences of implementing the *normalization* principle (Nirje, 1970; Wolfensberger, 1972). In this example, he points out the discrepancy between a social *principle*, suggesting that people with and without disabilities should live their lives in "integrated" settings, and the *reality* that people with disabilities sometimes *want* to engage in segregated activities. The specific examples that he cites are *Special Olympics* and the *People First* organization, both of which involve the congregation of people with disabilities. Can these activities be wrong, he speculates, simply because they do not conform with the "principle of normalization," when there is obvious evidence that those who participate in these organizations do so with obvious enthusiasm and enjoyment?

If personal choice is, in fact, a *sine qua non* for the subjective approach to determining quality of life, we must assume that the ability to choose is available to everyone. Rosen (1986) raises this question from the perspective of people with mental retardation who may have difficulty in conceptualizing alternatives as a precursor to making choices. He suggests that we resolve this dilemma by teaching people how to choose, but acknowledges that we may still be left with a problem if we believe that someone for whom we are responsible may be making a "unwise" choice.

Even Edgerton (1990) acknowledges this dilemma with the following caveat:

It is clear that we cannot abdicate all responsibility for setting limits to an individual's freedom of choice. We cannot tolerate risks to the public health, nor can we ignore some kinds of self-injurious behavior, and we must obviously draw the line at behaviors that harm others. But few instances are as clear-cut as these (p. 152).

Perhaps Edgerton is correct in identifying anti-social and self-injurious choices as being most clearly unacceptable. When thinking about "basic needs," however, where does one draw the line? Remembering Edgerton's earlier anecdote, is it proper to stand by silently and know that someone is being exposed to AIDS, especially if that person does not understand the consequences of his behavior? Even in less dangerous situations, are these certain "universal needs", such as food, clothing and housing, that everyone is *entitled* to, whether or not that person actively chooses to address such needs?

The question of entitlement was addressed directly by both Rosen (1986) and Edgar (1987), who assert that everyone is entitled to some "minimum" quality of life. To the extent that this involves the acquisition of resources, entitlement is obviously a political issue as well as an issue surrounding the definition of quality of life. At the political level, only governments can guarantee such basic necessities as food, clothing and shelter to an entire population. Edgar (1987) was actually fairly cynical about the possibility of such "entitlements" in a capitalist society such as ours.

At the conceptual level, as it pertains to a definition of quality of life, the definition of entitlement becomes somewhat difficult to ascertain. Perhaps few would argue with the most basic of human needs. But when does one person's nomination of an entitlement become another person's nomination of a personal option? Edgar's (1987) own list of entitlements makes the issue clear. He suggests that everyone is entitled to a quality of life that includes the following 7 domains: (a) safety, (b) pleasantness, (c) friends and companions, (d) self-esteem, (e) fun, (f) accomplishments/productivity (in whatever we do), and (g) excitement. It is not likely that everyone's list of entitlements would be identical to Edgar's list.

Another dichotomy that has emerged in the quality-of-life literature is the difference between personal needs and social expectations (Goode, 1990; Parmenter, 1988). Goode even builds this distinction into his definition of quality of life, as cited above. His model includes several components, including:

1. personal needs, mediated by the availability of environmental resources;
2. social expectations, mediated by the presence or absence of individual abilities; and
3. quality-of-life goals, mediated by *both* individual goals and social expectations.

A possible example within this model (which is mine, not his) might include the following parts, which in some ways resemble a syllogism:

1. If a person has a *need* to work and there are appropriate job *opportunities* in the person's environment; and
2. If the social milieu of the person *expects* that person to work and the person either has or could have the *ability* to work; then
3. It is appropriate to seek the necessary resources in the community and cultivate the necessary abilities in the person; and
4. It is appropriate to measure vocational outcomes as one "objective" indicator of that person's quality of life.

Within this example, social expectations serve as an influence on the choices that are made by an individual. Parmenter (1988) even broadens the definition of this type of influence to include any societal "condition," such as level of general unemployment, that might influence a person's choice of what to pursue in order to enhance quality of life.

One final dichotomy that we find within the quality-of-life literature is the distinction between *personal intervention* and *social policy development* as potential uses for quality-of-life information. Both purposes have been proposed frequently, and it seems obvious that the former is served best when we view quality of life from a personal perspective, and the latter is served best when we view quality of life from a societal perspective. How, then, can we combine the 2 perspectives into an integrated definitional and procedural framework? I propose the following strategy as a first step in this direction.

Strategy for conceptual integration. Let us begin by assuming that there is value in discriminating between individual and societal perspectives on quality of life. From an individual perspective, *personal choice* is the basic principle. If one chooses any particular outcome, such as employment, then the measurement of that outcome is relevant. Such measurement can be both objective (e.g., is the person employed?) and subjective (e.g., is the person satisfied with the job?). The purpose of measuring quality of life from an individual perspective is to help *that person* to establish as high a quality of life as is possible. This may require teaching the person how to choose, and in some cases (hopefully not many), making some choices for he person or restricting some choices if they are anti-social or self-injurious. The quality-of-life information that is collected should be used for several purposes, including (a) individualized planning, (b) monitoring individual outcomes, and (c) modifying interventions until successful outcomes are achieved.

From a societal perspective, *social norms* are the most meaningful frame of reference. The goal is to identify socially desirable goals for *groups* of people, as a whole, acknowledging that conformity with such norms *may not be appropriate for any given individual* within the norm group. The starting point for a taxonomy of norms would be the identification of presumed "basic social entitlements". Information collected on representative samples should then be used to determine how well, or poorly, the social norms are being experienced by groups of people who are represented by the samples. Interestingly enough, both "objective" and "subjective" measures are appropriate for this purpose. For example, the attainment of social norms in employment can be measured both by objective indices of employment status and by subjective indices of job satisfaction. As this type of knowledge is accumulated, appropriate recommendations should emerge concerning desirable changes in public policy and program development.

Linkage between the 2 perspectives. Even after acknowledging that any given individual's choices with respect to quality of life may appropriately deviate from general societal norms, the question still remains concerning how to identify such norms for the majority of people within any given reference group. Our proposed starting point is to identify "presumed basic social entitlements" for a taxonomy of such norms. But how do we know that any given list is appropriate?

The concept of "social validity" (Romer and Heller, 1983; Walker and Calkins, 1986) may provide a useful framework for answering this question. The process would begin by identifying those quality-of-life domains that have been proposed most frequently to be included in a taxonomy of entitlements. The list could even be augmented with 1 or more "novel" domains that have been proposed by someone, with convincing argumentation, to be included as indices of quality of life. Once the list has been determined, each domain identified would then be evaluated in terms of its *importance* as a component of quality of life. The evaluators would be members of an appropriate reference group, which in our case would be adolescents and young adults with disabilities as well as their parents and possibly other members of their families. If such research were undertaken with multiple samples, over time we would develop a consensual model identifying appropriate societal norms.

Specific content domains. As mentioned toward the beginning of this paper, the definition of quality of life for special education students in transition began in the narrowest possible way, with a focus entirely on employment (Will, 1984). I suggested an expansion of this focus to include residential and personal/social domains in addition to employment, and also to examine personal satisfaction as part of the mix (Halpern, 1985; 1989). Although a step in the right direction, these early efforts were not nearly sufficient in identifying the complexity of quality of life. The new special education legislation (P.L. 101–476), however, sets the stage for a much broader interpretation of quality of life. After reviewing an extensive amount of follow-along literature and thinking about possible taxonomies over the years with colleagues, we have developed a proposed list of content domains that should be considered when attempting to understand quality of life for special education students in transition. With full awareness that the list may still be incomplete from the perspective of others, we offer it as a point of departure for social validation research.

When one examines the various taxonomies that have been proposed for classifying quality-of-life outcomes, 3 basic domains of outcome are almost always represented. These include:

1. physical and material well-being;
2. performance of a variety of adult roles; and
3. a sense of personal fulfillment

We have identified 15 types of outcome that fall into these 3 domains and seem to capture much of the content that is mentioned often in the quality-of-life literature.

Physical and material well-being. The types of outcome that are represented in this domain seem to include what Edgar (1987) and Rosen (1986) have described as entitlements. Unless these outcomes are achieved, at least to some reasonable extent, it would be very difficult to achieve the outcomes that are listed in the other two domains. Four such "basic" outcomes have been identified as falling into this first domain:

1. physical and mental health
2. food, clothing and lodging
3. safety from harm
4. financial security

Performance of adult roles. The next level of outcome includes the many ways in which a person can interact with his or her environment. Terms that have been used to describe such outcomes include community adjustment, community integration, independent living, and interdependent living. We have identified 8 types of outcome that seem to fit well into this domain:

1. mobility and community access
2. vocation, career, employment
3. leisure and recreation
4. personal relationships and social networks
5. educational attainment
6. spiritual fulfillment
7. citizenship (e.g., voting)
8. social responsibility (e.g., doesn't break laws)

Personal fulfillment. As argued eloquently by Taylor and Bogdan (1990) and Edgerton (1990), a sense of personal fulfillment does not always correspond to the achievement of success, as commonly defined, in the various adult roles listed above. This dimension of quality of life is entirely person-centered, even though it is influenced by interactions with one's environment. Three types of outcome have been described in this domain:

1. happiness
2. satisfaction
3. a sense of general well-being

Edgerton (1990) discusses the differences between these 3 outcomes fairly succinctly. Happiness is a transient state of affect, usually governed by events that are happening at the moment. Satisfaction refers to behavior patterns and events over a longer period of time, but is often specific to a given adult role. For example, one can be very unsatisfied at work but highly satisfied with personal and social relationships. General well-being is the most durable of the outcomes, and implies an enduring sense of satisfaction with the quality of one's life, almost irrespective of the events and conditions that lead to happiness or situation-specific satisfaction. Edgerton labels this last outcome "temperament" and suggests that it has been highly influential in determining the quality of life for those people whom he studied over many years. The term "temperament" may be too restricting, however, implying that general well-being is primarily affective in nature. A broader conceptualization that includes cognitive and motivational dimensions of well-being is captured in the literature by other terms such as *self-concept* and *self-esteem* (Coopersmith, 1967).

Summary. Three major programs have emerged in the United States over the past 30 years to address the needs of special education students as they are completing their secondary school education and are preparing to assume roles as young adults in their communities. The first of these programs, called cooperative work-study programs, began in the 1960's and focused on the needs of students with mild mental retardation. The second program, called career education, began in the 1970's and addressed the career development needs of all students, with and without disabilities. The third program, called transition, began in the 1980's and focused entirely on the needs of students with disabilities.

An underlying theme within all 3 programs was uncertainty and unclarity on the ultimate goals being addressed by the programs. Focusing always on employment as an intended outcome, the question arose constantly as to whether or not the desired outcomes should be extended to include other important dimensions of quality of life. These broader needs were always acknowledged, even when it was not clear what the program's responsibilities should be in addressing these needs.

As we move into the 1990's, the special education legislation in the United States (P.L. 101–467) clearly requires a broader mandate to examine multiple dimensions of quality of life as programs are developed and implemented for students with disabilities. Our analysis of the quality-of-life literature suggests that such an effort should address at least 15 content areas in 3 broad domains: physical and material well-being, performance of adult roles, and personal fulfillment. We turn next to an analysis of the follow-up and follow-along literature in secondary special education in order to examine the quality of life that has been experienced by school leavers with disabilities.

FOLLOW-UP AND FOLLOW-ALONG RESEARCH

In 1975, the United States Congress passed Public Law 94–142 which guaranteed a "free and appropriate" public school education for all students with disabilities. Since the passage of this law, a number of follow-up and follow-along studies have been conducted in order to attempt to evaluate the impact of the law on the lives of people with disabilities who have gone through the school system. Several reviews of this literature have recently been published, including a methodological review (Halpern, 1990) and a review of findings (Chadsey-Rusch *et al.*, 1991). In this section of the present paper, the research findings will be summarized briefly, the structure of the findings will be juxtaposed with the quality-of-life model presented above, and a general model of transition programming will be proposed to structure both research and program development in the future.

Overview of the research findings. Although numerous studies have been published during the past 15 years examining the school-to-community transition of youth with disabilities, there are sufficient methodological flaws in these studies to prevent a clear and convincing interpretation of the collective findings. As I discussed elsewhere (Halpern, 1990), these flaws include:

1. a strong tendency to employ a cross-sectional design (follow-up) rather than the more powerful longitudinal design (follow-along);
2. the use of inappropriate samples that neither generalize to a clearly defined population nor are of sufficient size to support the data analysis approach employed;
3. the use of inappropriate data collection techniques that produce low rates of return;
4. carelessness in the definition of variables, which produces findings that are difficult to interpret;
5. narrowness in the choice of outcome variables to examine, often focusing on employment alone; and
6. failure to articulate a model of transition to guide the overall structure of the investigation

Even in the presence of these methodological flaws, there are some findings that have emerged with sufficient frequency (Chadsey-Rusch *et al.*, 1991) that they are worthy of presentation to provide, at the very least, a sense of the problems and issues that must be addressed in future efforts to measure the impact of transition programs. The areas of post-school adjustment that have received the most attention include employment, residential adjustment and personal/social adjustment.

Employment. Many young adults with disabilities are unemployed. From the array of studies that have examined this area, it would appear that less than half of all youth with disabilities achieve full-time employment within 2 years of leaving school, which is 50 to 100 percent worse than findings that are available for youth without disabilities. Most of those who do find jobs receive little or no assistance in this endeavor from social or rehabilitation agencies. They find their jobs either by themselves or with the assistance of family or friends. Graduating from high school increases the likelihood of finding a job, as does the presence of good social skills. Deviant or maladaptive behavior, as might be expected, mitigates against finding or holding a job.

Residential adjustment. Most young adults with disabilities tend to live in the home of their parents for the first several years after leaving high school. This is also true for many school-leavers without disabilities, although to a lesser extent and for a shorter period of time. The underlying rationale seems to include both psychological and financial dependency. As was true in the case of employment, the presence of independent living skills and the absence of maladaptive behaviors are both fairly strong predictors of post-school residential independence.

Personal/social adjustment. Perhaps the most striking finding in this area is that young adults with disabilities tend to experience social isolation more frequently than their peers without disabilities. This is apparently true both during the last few years of high school and during the first several years out of school. When social isolation emerges during the years in school, this has often been identified as one of several major influences that causes students to drop out of school. Perhaps most disconcerting is the information that we are beginning to gather on criminal behavior. Preliminary findings suggest that youth with disabilities have higher arrest rates than their peers without disabilities, during the first several years out of school. This is especially true for students who have been labeled *emotionally disturbed* or *behavior disordered* during their school years.

Findings from a quality-of-life perspective. One of the findings that emerged from our methodological review of outcome studies (Halpern, 1990) was the overwhelming tendency of researchers to focus on employment as the sole or most important outcome of high school programs for students with disabilities. This is inconsistent, of course, with our quality-of-life perspective which suggests that we consider 3 broad domains and 15 specific content areas as a taxonomy of outcomes. Using this taxonomy as a frame of reference, we reviewed 41 follow-up and follow-along studies that have examined post-school outcomes of students with disabilities. These are listed as a subset within the references at the end of this paper. The selection criterion for review was that the study be published in a referred journal between 1975 and 1990, which covers essentially the Public Law 94–142 "era" of special education programs in the United States.

The purpose of this review was simply to determine *which domains and content areas* had been addressed within each study. We did not include "happiness" in this review, since this outcome was viewed as being too transient and situation specific to be properly included in the methodological designs of most follow-up and follow-along studies. The remaining 14 content areas were examined, and the findings are presented in Table I below.

Not surprisingly, all of the studies reported findings that pertained to career and employment. Perhaps because of its relationship to employment, financial security was also reported by approximately three-quarters of the studies. Educational attainment, most often from the singular perspective of graduating or dropping out, was reported in slightly more than half the studies. The only other area that was addressed by nearly half of the studies was personal relationships/social networks.

If we are to take seriously a quality-of-life model as a frame of reference for transition programs, we will obviously need to do a better job of attending to the various dimensions of quality of life. Given the theoretical concerns addressed above, perhaps the most glaring omission from many of the studies is the "personal fulfillment" domain. Without this personal perspective, one might argue that the other domains lose much of their significance.

Even if we are more careful about collecting information about personal fulfillment, the data in Table I suggest that we will still have to convince people that it is important to collect information in a variety of underrepresented and unrepresented content areas, if we want to examine quality of life in its most complete sense. We should also be examining, from a research perspective, the social validity of all the

TABLE I

Quality-of-Life Domains and Content Areas Addressed by 41 Follow-Up Studies

Domain	Content Area	Number of Times Used	Percent of Times Used
Physical and Material Well-Being	Physical and mental health	6	15%
	Food, clothing, lodging	10	24%
	Safety from harm	2	5%
	Financial security	31	76%
Performance of Adults Roles	Mobility, community access	9	22%
	Career and employment	41	100%
	Leisure and recreation	10	24%
	Relationships, social networks	18	44%
	Educational attainment	23	56%
	Spiritual fulfillment	0	0%
	Citizenship	0	0%
	Social responsibility	6	15%
Personal Fulfillment	Satisfaction	13	32%
	General well-being	5	12%

domains and content areas, in order to determine if the current level of representation is or is not appropriate.

A general model for transition programs. Outcome domains, as important as they are, comprise only one component of a general model of transition programs. A more complete model must also encompass program antecedents and program procedures that are relevant to transition outcomes. The amount of time captured under the umbrella of "transition" is obviously somewhat arbitrary. Some people have argued (Clark, 1979) that "career education" should begin when children are very young. At the other end of the continuum, it is almost impossible to determine when post-school "transition" has ended and other conceptual frameworks become more meaningful for addressing quality of life. As a minimal effort in model development, we suggest that the transition period should encompass the last year or two in school and the first year or two out of school.

If such a model were adopted, there are 6 types of information that would need to be gathered and analyzed in order to understand the model:

1. client and community demographic information
2. school services received
3. school outcomes achieved
4. quality of life while in school
5. post-school services received
6. quality of life after leaving school

Information within the first 4 domains should be gathered while the student is still in school. Information within the last 2 domains should be gathered (preferably at several time intervals) after the student has left school.

The 6 domains just identified serve 2 purposes within a research model. The first purpose is simply to describe the status of people from appropriate samples with respect to relevant variables within each domain. The second purpose is to understand the paths of influence between variables within each domain. Thinking of this second purpose, for example, one might be interested in understanding the relative impact of type of disability (Domain 1) and independent vocational skills attained (Domain 3) on whether or not the student had a well-paying job after school (Domain 4). The potential paths of influential that seem especially worthy of exploration are illustrated in Figure 2 below.

The implementation of the research model implied in Figure 2 begins with the specification of variables to be included and measured in each of the 6 domains. This is an extremely important step in the process, since the variables that are included for eventual measurement provide the "de facto" operational version of the model. Since most of the 41 studies reviewed above did not include a conceptual model as a frame

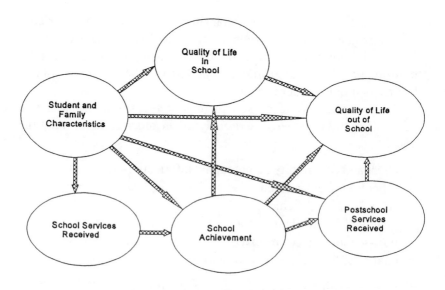

Fig. 2.   Basic follow-along conceptual model.

of reference for designing the study, it is not at all evident how the important decisions concerning variable selection were made.

Using the model in Figure 2 as a frame of reference, researchers at the University of Oregon have developed a follow-along strategy for conducting research on transition programs (Benz and Halpern, 1992; Halpern, 1990). The strategy is currently being implemented and evaluated in 3 states: Oregon, Nevada and Arizona. The operational development of the strategy was facilitated by a set of "research questions" that were articulated within each of the 6 major domains of the model. Several examples of these questions are presented in Table II below.

The articulation of these research questions serves several purposes within the Oregon Follow-Along Strategy. At an operational level, the questions have provided a "blue print" for the construction of items that appear in the data collection instruments. These items, in turn, provide the building blocks for he construction of variables to be included in the data analyses. By carefully referencing item construction to research questions and domains of interest, it is possible to examine regularly the

TABLE II

Examples of Research Questions From Each of the Six Follow-Along Domains

Domain	Research Question
Student and family characteristics	1. What is the basic structure of families being served (e.g., single parent or two parents, number of siblings)?
	2. What is the socioeconomic status of families being served?
School services needed and received	1. What kinds of vocational instruction do students with disabilities need and what instruction do they receive in high school?
	2. To what extent are students with disabilities satisfied with their school program?
School achievement and post school needs	1. How well are students with disabilities prepared in basic independent living skills?
	2. What proportion of students with disabilities graduate, drop out, or "age out" from high school?
Quality of life while in school	1. What types of friendships and intimate relationships are experience by students with disabilities?
	2. What proportion of students with disabilities experience social problems, such as drug abuse, being victimized by others, or incarceration?
Post-school services needed and received	1. What are the primary referral procedures utilized by school leavers with disabilities in their attempt to access services?
	2. What proportion of school leavers with disabilities received post-school services, and what kinds of services did they receive?
Quality of life out of school	1. What level of financial security is achieved by school leavers with disabilities, and what sources do they rely upon for their income?
	2. What proportion of school leavers with disabilities live independently or semi-independently in their communities?

rationale for including or excluding any given item for the final form of the instruments that are developed.

The research questions also provide a heuristic device for presenting findings back to intended users. One of the complaints frequently heard about follow-along research is that findings are often presented in a very laborious manner. It is not uncommon for such presentations to be offered as a large compendium of tables and graphs, resulting in a product that somewhat resembles a telephone book. When the research questions are used as a structure for presenting the research findings, however, the resulting products are short, succinct and focused on a particular concern that is represented by the question. Users of the information are encouraged to "pick and choose" the reports that may be of special interest to them.

The quality-of-life model described above, with its 3 domains and 15 content areas, plays an obvious and important role within the Oregon Follow-Along Strategy for conducting research on transition programs. As the 2 quality-of-life domains within the follow-along strategy (in-school and post-school) were operationalized, the domains and content areas within the quality-of-life model provided the blue print for item construction. Most, though not all, of the quality-of-life content areas were eventually represented in the instruments of the follow-along strategy.

If a follow-along strategy has been well structured and properly implemented, the findings are potentially very useful. In order for such utility to be realized, however, there must be clear and viable procedures in place for *attending* to the information when relevant *decisions* are being made. Two very different types of decisions can be influenced by follow-along information: program *planning* decisions for *individuals*, and program *development* decisions for *organizations*. These will both be addressed in the next and last section of this paper.

STRATEGIES FOR IMPROVING TRANSITION PROGRAMS

In the broad area of transition for students with disabilities, as in many other areas of life, decisions will be made whether or not they are influenced by a good understanding of the issues at hand. When making decisions of any kind, the procedures that people follow can range from well structured and explicit to poorly structured and implicit. The structure for decision-making in the area of transition for students with disabilities comes in part from the federal laws and regulations governing special education. This structure in itself, however, is insufficient. In order to be fully effective, it must be augmented with good information, such as that which is generated through an effective follow-along strategy, and good procedures for program planning and program development. These procedures can be either person-oriented or program-oriented.

Person-oriented decisions. Special education in the United States has been dominated during the past 15 years by a piece of federal legislation commonly referred to as Public Law 94–142. The essence of this law guarantees a *free and appropriate* public education for all children and youth with disabilities. Compliance with this law also requires that a "child study team" must develop an *individual education program* (IEP) for each student, and the IEP must be reviewed at least annually (Heward and Orlansky, 1991). The members of the child study team must include, at a minimum, (a) the child's teacher, (b) someone from the school other than the child's teacher, (c) the child's parents or guardian, and (d) the child, if appropriate.

A number of specific requirements have been specified for inclusion in any IEP. These requirements include:

1. a statement of the child's present levels of education performance in *all appropriate areas of potential instruction.*
2. a statement of annual goals for the next school year.
3. a statement of short-term instructional objectives that pertain to the annual goals.
4. a statement of specific educational services that are needed to achieve the goals and objectives.
5. a date when services will begin and a proposed length of services.
6. objective criteria for evaluating student achievement.
7. a list of those who are responsible for implementing the plan.

Follow-along information can obviously be quite relevant for several of these requirements, particularly the ones requiring documentation of present performance level and evaluation of student achievement.

The passage of Public Law 101–476 in 1990, which amends Public Law 94–142, was an important event in the legislative mandate for transition services. The proposed regulations for this act include the addition of several specific transition requirements for the IEP (Section 300.346):

The IEP shall include a statement of *needed transition services** for students beginning *no later than age 16** and annually thereafter (and when determined appropriate for the individual, beginning at 14 or younger), including when appropriate, a statement of the *interagency responsibilities** or linkages (or both) before the student leaves the school setting [*italics added].

In order to help with the implementation of this new requirement, the law also stipulates that 1 or more representatives of adult agencies should be added to the child study team, when appropriate.

The implementation of these new requirements will not be easy. As previous research has shown (Benz and Halpern, 1987; Edgar, 1987), many high school programs for students with disabilities do not presently address transition needs adequately. But the opportunities are there, and these opportunities will be highly reinforced by the new law. Our challenge is to develop good procedures for doing transition planning, and to use follow-along information both to guide the initial selection of goals and objectives, and to evaluate accomplishment of the goals and objectives. A good quality-of-life model should also play an important role in helping members of the IEP child study team to reflect carefully on *intended outcomes* during the process of developing transition programs.

Program-oriented decisions. An assumption that clearly underlies the IEP process is that programs and services are actually *available* and of sufficient *quality* to address effectively any given individual's transition needs. This assumption is rarely met in the real world. Instead, we are often faced with situations where a person's needs are evident and yet there are no programs or resources available to address those needs adequately. The planning that is needed in this type of situation is program development or "capacity" building (Heal *et al.*, 1990). In the area of secondary special education and transition programs, such capacity building is fairly complex because it involves the school system, the adult service system, the private sector (e.g., employers), and the interaction between all three. A *systems-change* model is needed in order to achieve such capacity building in an orderly and effective manner (A. Halpern *et al.*, 1992).

For the past 7 years, almost immediately following the announcement of the transition initiative by Madeleine Will (1984), we at the University of Oregon have been involved in the development, implementation and evaluation of such a systems-change model. When this effort first began, we identified 4 basic conditions that needed to be present in order for a systems-change model to work (Becklund and Haring, 1982; Hord *et al.*, 1987).

1. The model must be *guided* by a set of *program standards* which provide a rationale for change and a set of targets for guiding change.
2. The model must be *implemented* through a set of efficient and effective *procedures* which provide structure for the program improvement efforts of diverse stakeholders in local communities. These stakeholders include people with disabilities and their families, school personnel, adult agency personnel, and members of the general public such as employers.
3. The model must be *supported* by the provision of *training and technical assistance* to those who are responsible for implementing the mode.
4. The model must be *documented* with concise and effective *materials*, so that the program improvement efforts can be replicated efficiently and effectively.

The model that we developed incorporated each of these conditions, and is called the Community Transition Team Model (CTTM).

The content structure that undergirds all of the capacity-building procedures within the CTTM is a set of *program standards*. These standards emerged from a set of research efforts that were designed to identify unmet *program* needs in the broad area of secondary special education and transition programs (Benz and Halpern, 1986; Benz and Halpern, 1987; Halpern and Benz, 1987; Halpern, 1987). Six areas were identified, including (a) curriculum and instruction, (b) coordination and mainstreaming, (c) transition services, (d) documentation of student outcomes, (e) adult services, and (f) administrative support. The full description of these needs is found elsewhere (Halpern *et al.*, 1992).

The development of program standards involved a careful examination of the unmet needs that were found in each of the 6 areas mentioned above, followed by a "conversion" of the need statement into a program standard which, if achieved, would address the need satisfactorily. For example, one identified need was a paucity of suitable job placements for school leavers with disabilities, which was related, in part, to a lack of appropriate opportunities for vocational instruction while the students were still in school. This program need was translated into the following program standard: *Students with disabilities receive appropriate vocational instruction, which prepares them for jobs in their communities.* A total of 38 standards eventually emerged from this process. Examples within each of the 6 areas are found in Table III below.

The standards within the CTTM are used by *community* transition teams, as a starting point for their *program* building efforts in their local communities. These community teams are quite different from the many IEP teams that work with individual students. The community teams, which focus all of their attention of program development rather than planning for individuals, include as members the full array of people who are concerned about secondary special education and transition programs in their communities. This array of team members includes representatives of four groups: (1) people with disabilities and their families, (2) school personnel, (3) adult agency personnel, and (4) members of the general public such as employers. During the past 7 years, 38 teams throughout Oregon, ranging in size from 10 to 25 members, have participated in the development, implementation, evaluation and refinement of the CTTM.

The actual implementation of the CTTM is organized around a typical management-by-objectives paradigm. The model has 5 basic components: (1) team building, (2) needs assessment, (3) program planning, (4) program implementation and evaluation, and (5) repetition of the

TABLE III

Examples of Program Standards Within the Community Transition Team Model

Area of Need	Program Standard
Curriculum and instruction	1. Students with disabilities receive appropriate instruction in social/interpersonal skills, which prepares them to interact effectively with people in their communities.
	2. Procedures exist for placing students into an instructional program that is tailored to their individual needs.
Coordination and mainstreaming	1. Students with disabilities have opportunities to learn prerequisite skills that are needed to participate in regular academic programs.
	2. A process exists for enhancing program planning and administrative collaboration between special education and the regular vocational program.
Transition	1. Information exists on community services currently available for school leavers with disabilities.
	2. A process exists for enhancing collaboration between special education and relevant adult agencies.
Documentation	1. Procedures exist for evaluating the immediate impact of instruction in terms of student learning outcomes.
	2. Procedures exist for conducting systematic follow-along evaluations on the community adjustment of school leavers with disabilities.
Administrative support	1. Administrative procedures exist for using aides, volunteers, and job coaches effectively within secondary special education programs, both in the school and in the community.
	2. Appropriate in-service training is regularly provided to personnel who are responsible for secondary special education and transition programs.
Adult services and community resources	1. Sufficient service programs and community resources are available to meet the residential needs of young adults with disabilities.
	2. Sufficient service programs and community resources are available to meet the employment needs of young adults with disabilities.

cycle. Since needs assessment is the component that has potential link-age with follow-along information, this component will be described in detail here. A more complete description of all the procedures can be found elsewhere (Halpern *et al.*, 1992).

The needs assessment process begins as soon as a community team has been organized, using an instrument containing the standards that has been specifically designed for use within the CTTM (Halpern *et al.*, 1990). The purpose of the needs assessment is to identify a small number of standards from the complete set that are of "highest priority" to serve as goals for the transition team to address. The format of the needs assessment involves rating each standard along 2 dimensions: perceived value and current status. The following Likert scales are used to create the ratings:

Value

Critical	Important	Somewhat Useful	Not Important
3	2	1	0

Current Status

Completely Achieved	Mostly Achieved	Partially Achieved	Not Achieved
0	1	2	3

The total score for any given standard is the sum of the 2 ratings, which has a maximum value of 6. Any standard receiving a score of 6 would obviously be a candidate for selection as "high priority," since such a standard would be viewed as both critical and not achieved. The average scores over a group of respondents represent a collective perception of priorities.

The connection between follow-along information and this systems-change model lies in the ratings of current status. The information that is collected through the Oregon follow-along instruments is relevant to approximately 60 percent of the standards that structure the CTTM, namely, those that address student needs and student behaviors, as contrasted with those that address the needs and behaviors of teachers and administrators. If relevant follow-along information can be presented to the raters, in a format that is clear and concise, then raters will be able to use this information when they are forming their opinions about the adequacy of "current status" as it pertains to a given standard. The development of such linkage procedures between the follow-along and systems-change models is currently underway at the University of Oregon.

As mentioned above, the Community Transition Team Model has been under development in Oregon over the past 7 years. A number of supporting materials are available to assist in its implementation, including a manual of procedures for transition team leaders (Halpern et al., 1990), a manual of guidelines for facilitators (Benz et al., 1990) who work with a state network of team leaders, and a software system for implementing procedures and producing reports that are specified within the CTTM (Lindstrom et al., 1990). The model, in varying degrees, is currently being replicated or adapted in several other states including Nevada, Kansas, Arizona and New South Wales. Only parts of the model were adapted to fit into the Australian effort, which drew upon a variety of models and influences and ultimately developed a very original approach (Parmenter and Riches, 1990).

The network of transition teams in Oregon has achieved an impressive array of accomplishments thus far, which includes both tangible outcomes, such as the development of new instructional programs, and less tangible outcomes, such as the establishment of improved communication and collaboration among service providers in a local community. The following anecdote illustrates the kinds of outcomes that have been achieved by transition teams as they have implemented the Community Transition Team Model. The example, which has also been reported elsewhere (Halpern et al., 1992) is a curriculum development effort that emerged from one of the first transition teams to participate in the Oregon project.

Their effort started with an idea for collaboration between a special education teacher and a business education teacher who were participating on the transition team. The special education teacher wanted a project that would provide opportunities for his students to gain work experience, become more involved in learning functioning independent living skills, expand their friendships, and enhance their self-esteem. The business education teacher wanted a project that would give his students experience in defining and setting up a small business.

A program called "snack attack" was conceived to meet both needs. Special education students would operate a business in school that provided mid-morning snacks to all students in the school. Business education students would develop a plan for the business, including such areas as purchasing supplies, packaging, marketing, distribution, and managing inventory.

Weekly program operations included soliciting orders for 7 different kinds of snacks from each home room in the school, and maintaining sufficient inventory to accommodate the orders. The next steps included packaging and delivering the orders to each home room representative, and then collecting funds, receipts, and unsold inventory at the end of the week. Literally buckets of cash were collected, which then required counting the funds received, reconciling inventory sold with funds received, and depositing funds in a bank account.

The immediate benefits of the program included intense involvement of the special education students in a project of great interest, as well as a variety of opportunities to interact meaningfully with regular students: both those in the business education class, and the "customers" in the business enterprise. But the benefits were only beginning to accrue as the program got underway.

Within several months, profits were approaching $700 per week, and the students had a problem: what to do with all their money. After much discussion they decided that they would rent an apartment nearby, to provide a good learning environment for practising a variety of independent living skills. This involved negotiating a lease with a landlord, fixing up and cleaning up the house, negotiating an agreement for electricity and water from the local utilities company, and eventually practising cooking and home maintenance skills.

Still there was money left over. Next, they decided to present a gift back to the school, to be used for any worthwhile project designated by the general student body. Still there was money left over. So they decided to make a gift to a worthwhile community organization, and eventually they chose a program for battered women.

It takes a lot of projects to spend $700 per week, and there was more to be done. The students eventually decided that they would pay for expenses so that the entire class could attend the annual meeting of the Oregon Vocational Association and present their program to interested parents and professionals. They prepared a video tape to present visually some important parts of their program, and each student read (or memorized) a script to provide an audio accompaniment to key parts of the visual presentation. During their free time, like other conventioneers, they kicked up their heels a bit and had a grand time enjoying themselves.

Throughout this whole process, a tremendous esprit de corps emerged, accompanied by a growing sense of self-worth and self-esteem. Who would have thought that so much would grow from the hatching of a simple idea!

SUMMARY

During the past 3 decades, the educational and community adjustment needs of adolescents and young adults with disabilities in the United States have been addressed through several school-based programs. These programs have come to be known as *work-study, career education*, and *transition* programs. Only the transition programs remain in operation today.

The goals of all 3 programs, although somewhat multi-dimensional, have tended to focus inordinately on employment, ignoring or minimizing other important aspects of quality of life. A broader and more comprehensive approach to outcomes is clearly needed, which from our perspective would include 3 major domains: physical and mental well-being, performance of valued adult roles, and personal fulfillment. Fifteen more specific content areas within these 3 domains have also been proposed for guiding both research and program development that pertains to adolescents and young adults with disabilities. The validity of this conceptual structure should continue to be evaluated through social validation research.

A follow-along strategy has been proposed for linking the research and program development efforts. This linkage must occur both in the transition plans that are developed for individual students and in the program development efforts that occur in local communities in order to develop capacity to address the needs of individuals. Models for doing both types of planning were presented and illustrated.

Within this broad context for potential change, there are several specific directions that should be followed if we are to enhance the quality of life for students and school-leavers with disabilities who are in transition from high school settings into new roles as young adults in their communities. There are 4 specific recommendations that I believe are worthy of special consideration: (1) enhancing self-determination, (2) developing a full array of instructional programs, (3) enhancing inclusive instructional environments, and (4) improving the array of community resources that are available.

Enhancing self-determination. When a person is labeled as having a disability, it is not uncommon for parents, service providers and family members to regard such people as being unable to learn how to take responsibility for their own lives. Such an attitude is especially prevalent when the disability being considered is a cognitive disability. When such attitudes are overly and inappropriately protective of the person with a disability, the consequence is to diminish that person's ability and opportunity for assuming fully adult roles in the community.

A school setting does not necessarily provide students with good opportunities to learn self-determination skills.   Conformity with existing instructional programs, largely determined by teachers and school administrators, often excludes opportunities to genuinely explore options and take responsibility for choices. Students are not expected to make plans, either for their present or their future lives.

As described above, the Individuals with Disabilities Education Act of 1990 (PL 101–476) has articulated the requirement that individualized education plans (IEP's) *must include transition planning* for *all students with disabilities above the age of 16.* One way or another, this requirement will be addressed in United States schools over the next several years. This requirement for transition planning within the IEP process provides an opportunity, but not a guarantee, for increasing the ability of students with disabilities to make wise decisions about their future plans after leaving school, as well as the programs and services they need while in school that will lay a good foundation for the future. If this planning process is to guided and influenced by *student self-determination*, however, a strategy must be carefully developed, implemented and evaluated to help students become empowered to play such an assertive role within the IEP process.

Although IEP requirements have been in existence since 1975, since the passage of Public Law 94–142, the implementation of these requirements in individual school districts has often occurred in a somewhat perfunctory manner. Teachers have usually assumed major responsibility for structuring IEP meetings, with students and parents often taking a very passive role in the process. Such an approach is clearly undesirable from the perspective of helping students and families to assume ever increasing amounts of responsibility for determining their own educational goals and objectives. The need for such self-determination is especially great as issues pertaining to transition from school into the adult community begin to assume increasing levels of importance in the lives of students and their families.

The achievement of student self-determination with the IEP process requires that the following 3 conditions must be achieved:

1. students must have an image of their long-range goals, an awareness of resources that are available to help them reach their goals, and a sense of *empowerment* that they are capable of assuming responsibility for such decisions;
2. students must have access to useful information about their own strengths and weaknesses, and they must accept *ownership* of that information as reflecting their own *self-evaluation*, rather than externally imposed evaluations; and
3. students must have a *workable strategy* for using this information *themselves* in the development, implementation, modification and evaluation of their own transition plans.

If programs are developed that address these 3 conditions, student self-determination will be enhanced which, in turn, will enhance student potential for enjoying an enhanced quality of life.

Developing instructional programs. Planning, however, is not enough, even is such planning is driven by opportunities to learn and practice self-determination. There must be in place an array of appropriate *options* from which students can choose those that are relevant for his or her long and short-range goals.

The history of program opportunities for students with disabilities, as described above, has tended over the decades to focus too much on traditional academics at the expense of providing instruction that might enhance employment, independent living, and the acquisition of personal and social skills. Efforts to expand opportunities in these areas, such as those that have emerged from the implementation of *Community Transition Team Model*, represent a fruitful counter-trend that has emerged during the last decade. If we continue to encourage this type of development, students will choose more appropriate options for learning opportunities which, in turn, will enhance their quality of life.

Enhancing inclusive instructional environments. To an extent, quality of life is denigrated when people are *forced* to segregate themselves from the mainstream of their cultural milieu. The history of special education in the United States has often included such forced segregation of students with disabilities into "special classes", totally removed from the general education environment. There have, however, been counter trends that began with the "mainstreaming" initiatives of the 1970's, progressed to the "regular education initiative" of the 1980's, and currently are expressed as the "full inclusion" models of the 1990's. Each of these initiatives or models has focused, one way or another, on providing opportunities for people with disabilities to receive their instruction in regular education environments, along with and along side of students without disabilities.

I mentioned above how such initiatives can sometimes go too far, forbidding people the right to *choose* to segregate for certain purposes, such as Special Olympics or the People First organization. These exceptions aside, it is clearly desirable *to provide opportunities* for special education students to receive their education in the company of regular education students and teachers. Such experiences help to break down inappropriate stereotypes about disability and provide opportunities for social relationships to develop that would otherwise hardly ever occur. When this occurs, the quality of life for students *both with and without disabilities* is very likely to be enhanced.

Improving the array of community resources. The ultimately desired outcomes of a life imbued with quality are reflected in the taxonomy presented above in Table I. As this taxonomy suggests, the enjoyment of a high quality of life includes physical and mental well being, the performance of chosen adult roles, and a resulting sense of personal fulfillment. The achievement of such goals can only be partially achieved as a consequence of effective high school programs. A great deal will also depend on the availability and quality of resources that can be found within the adult communities into which school-leavers will move during the transition years.

There are at least 4 very different types of resources that are potentially available within communities. The first might be described as the basic structure of the community, including such things as the availability of housing, transportation, goods and services. The second type of resource includes agencies and services that are available to help people access what is available within the basic structure of their communities. Such services can be either generically available to anyone or specifically designed to address the needs of people with disabilities. The third type of resource includes the network of family and friends that each person has to provide context and color to his or her life activities. The fourth type of resource includes community organizations, such as churches and social groups, that provide additional opportunities for people to become integrated into their communities. One's ability to access these various community resources has a profound effect on his or her quality of life.

In summary, there are many paths that different people follow as they pursue their own dreams and achieve, to greater and lesser extents, a high quality of life. The essential requirement for making this journey successfully is the ability to exercise choice and self-determination effectively. While in school, students with disabilities need opportunities a very broad range of instructional programs, responsive to their individual needs and provided, when appropriate, in an inclusive environment that breaks down forced segregation from students without disabilities. Once out of school, attention must also be given to helping school-leavers with disabilities to access those community resources that are still needed in order to support the enjoyment of a high quality of life.

REFERENCES

Becklund, J. D. and N. G. Haring: 1982, Strategies for Change in Special Education: Maintaining and Transferring Effective Innovations (University of Washington Press, Seattle, WA).

Benz, M. and A. Halpern: 1986, 'Vocational preparation for high school students with mild disabilities: A statewide study of administrator, teacher, and parent perceptions', Career Development for Exceptional Individuals 9, pp. 3–15.

Benz, M. and A. Halpern: 1987, 'Transition services for secondary students with mild disabilities: A statewide perspective', Exceptional Children 53, pp. 507–514.

Benz, M., L. Lindstrom, A. Halpern and R. Rotherstrom: 1990, Community Transition Team Model: Facilitator's Manual (University of Oregon, Eugene, OR).

Brolin, D.: 1983, 'Career education: Where do we go from here?', Career Development for Exceptional Individuals 6, pp. 3–14.

Brown, R., M. Bayer and C. FacFarlane: 1988, 'Quality of life amongst handicapped adults', in R. Brown (ed.), Quality of Life for Handicapped People (Croom Helm, London).

Cegelka, P.: 1979, 'Career education', in M. Epstein and D. Cullinan (eds.), Special Education for Adolescents: Issues and Perspectives (Charles E. Merrill, Columbus, OH), pp. 155–184.

Chadsey-Rusch, J., F. Rusch and M. O'Reilly: 1991, 'Transition from schools to integrated communities', Remedial and Special Education 12, pp. 23–33.

Clark, G.: 1979, Career Education for the Handicapped in the Elementary Classroom (Love Publishing Company, Denver).

Coopersmith, S.: 1967, The Antecedents of Self-Esteem (W. H. Freeman and Company, San Francisco).

Edgar, E.: 1987, 'Secondary programs in special education: Are many of them justifiable?', Exceptional Children 53, pp. 555–561.

Edgar, E.: 1987, Early Morning Thoughts on the Quality of Life (University of Washington, Seattle, WA), unpublished manuscript.

Edgerton, R.: 1990, 'Quality of life from a longitudinal research perspective', in R. Schalock and M. Begab (eds.), Quality of Life: Perspectives and Issues (American Association on Mental Retardation, Washington, D.C.)

Goode, D.: 1990, 'Thinking about and discussing quality of life', in R. Schalock and M. Begab (eds.), Quality of Life: Perspectives and Issues (American Association on Mental Retardation, Washington, D.C.).

Halpern, A.: 1993, 'General unemployment and vocational opportunities for EMR individuals', American Journal of Mental Deficiency 80, pp. 81–89.

Halpern, A.: 1974, 'Work-study programs for the mentally retarded: An overview', in P. Browning (ed.), Mental Retardation: Rehabilitation and Counselling (Charles C Thomas, Springfield, IL).

Halpern, A.: 1985, 'Transition: A look at the foundations', Exceptional Children 51, pp. 479–486.

Halpern, A.: 1987, 'Characteristics of a quality program', in C. Warger and B. Weiner (eds.), Secondary Special Education: A Guide to Promising Public School Programs (Council for Exceptional Children, Reston, VA), pp. 25–55.

Halpern, A.: 1989, 'A systematic approach to transition programming for adolescents and young adults with disabilities', Australia and New Zealand Journal of Developmental Disabilities 15, pp. 1–13.

Halpern, A.: 1990, 'A methodological review of follow-up and follow-along studies tracking school leavers in special education', Career Development for Exceptional Individuals 13, pp. 13–28.

Halpern, A.: 1992, 'Transition: Old wine in new bottles', Exceptional Children 58, pp. 202–212.

Halpern, A. and M. Benz: 1987, 'A statewide examination of secondary special education for students with mild disabilities: Implications for the high school curriculum', Exceptional Children 54, pp. 122–129.

Halpern, A., M. Benz and L. Lindstrom: 1992, 'A systems change approach to improving secondary special education and transition programs at the local community level', Career Development for Exceptional Individuals 15, pp. 109–120.

Halpern, A., L. Lindstrom and M. Benz: 1990, Community Transition Team Model: Needs Assessment Instrument (University of Oregon, Eugene, OR).

Halpern, A., D. Nelson, L. Lindstrom and M. Benz: 1990, Community Transition Team Model: Team Leader's Manual (University of Oregon, Eugene, OR).

Heal, L. W., J. I. Copher and F. R. Rusch: 1990, 'Inter-agency agreements (IAAs) among agencies responsible for the transition education of students with handicaps for secondary schools to post-secondary settings', Career Development for Exceptional Individuals 13, pp. 121–127.

Heward, W. and M. Orlansky: 1991, Exceptional Children (4th ed.) (Merrill Publishing Company, Columbus, OH).

Hord, S. M., W. L. Rutherford, L. Huling-Austin and G. E. Hall: 1987, Taking Charge of Change (Association for Supervision and Curriculum Development, Alexandria, VA).

Hoyt, K.: 1982, 'Career education: Beginning of the end, or a new beginning?', Career Development for Exceptional Individuals 5, pp. 3–12.

Kolstoe, O. and R. Frey: 1965, A High School Work-study Program for Mentally Subnormal Students (Southern Illinois University Press, Carbondale, IL).

Lindstrom, L., W. Ard, M. Benz and A. Halpern: 1990, Community Transition Team Model: Management Information System Manual (University of Oregon, Eugene, OR).

MacFarlane, C., R. Brown and M. Bayer: 1989, 'Rehabilitation programmes study: Quality of life', in R. Brown, M. Bayer and C. MacFarlane (eds.), Rehabilitation Programmes: Performance and Quality of Life of Adults with Developmental Handicaps (Lugus Productions Ltd., Toronto).

Nirje, B.: 1970, 'The normalization principle: Implications and comments', Journal of Mental Subnormality 16, pp. 62–70.

Parmenter, T.: 1988, 'An analysis of the dimensions of quality of life for people with physical disabilities', in R. I. Brown (ed.), Quality of Life for Handicapped People: A Series in Rehabilitation Education (Croom Helm, London).

Parmenter, T. and V. Riches: 1990, Establishing individual transition planning for students with disabilities within the New South Wales Department of School Education (Macquarie University, Sydney), unpublished manuscript.

Position paper on career education: 1978 (Council for Exceptional Children, Reston, VA).

Romer, D. and T. Heller: 1983, 'Social adaptation of mentally retarded adults in community settings: A social ecological approach', Applied Research in Mental Retardation 4, pp. 303–314.

Rosen, M.: 1986, 'Quality of life for persons with mental retardation: A question of entitlement', Mental Retardation 24, pp. 365–366.

Schalock,R.: 1990, 'Attempts to conceptualize and measure quality of life', in R. Schalock and M. Begab (eds.), Quality of Life: Perspectives and Issues (American Association on Mental Retardation, Washington, D.C.).

Taylor, S. and R. Bogdan: 1990, 'Quality of life and the individual's perspective', in R. Schalock and M. Begab (eds.), Quality of Life: Perspectives and Issues (American Association on Mental Retardation, Washington, D.C.).

Walker, H. and C. Calkins: 1986, 'The role of social competence in the community adjustment of persons with developmental disabilities: Process and outcomes', Journal of Remedial and Special Education 7, pp. 46–53.

Will, M.: 1984, OSERS Programming for the Transition of Youth with Disabilities: Bridges From School to Working Life (Office of Special Education and Rehabilitative Services, Washington, D.C.).

Wolfensberger, W.: 1972, Normalization: The Principle of Normalization in Human Services (National Institute on Mental Retardation, Toronto).

FOLLOW-UP STUDIES REFERENCED IN TABLE I

Affleck, J. Q., E. Edgar, P. Levine and L. Kortering: 1990, 'Postschool status of students classified as mildly mentally retarded, learning disabled, or nonhandicapped: Does it get better with time?', Education and Training in Mental Retardation 25, pp. 315–324.

Brolin, D., R. Durand, K. Kromer, and P. Muller: 1975, 'Post-school adjustment of educable retarded students', Education and Training of the Mentally Retarded 10, pp. 144–149.

Bullis, M., B. Bull, B. Johnson, P. Johnson and Kittrell: 1990, School-to-community Transition Experiences of Hearing Impaired Adolescents and Young Adults in the Northwest (Teaching Research Division, Western Oregon State College, Monmouth, OR).

Clemmons, D. C. and C. B. Dodrill: 1983, 'Vocational outcomes of high school students with epilepsy', Journal of applied Rehabilitation Counselling 14, pp. 49–53.

DeBettencourt, L. U., N. Zigmond and H. Thornton: 1989, 'Follow-up of postsecondary-age rural learning disabled graduates and dropouts', Exceptional Children 56, pp. 40–49.

Edgar, E.: 1988, 'Employment as an outcome for mildly handicapped students: Current status and future directions', Focus on Exceptional Children 21, pp. 1–8.

Fafard, M. and P. A. Haubrich: 1981, 'Vocational and social adjustment of learning disabled young adults: A followup study', Learning Disability Quarterly 4, pp. 122–130.

Fardig, D. B., R. F. Algozzine, S. E. Schwartz, J. W. Hensel and D. L. Westling: 1985, 'Postsecondary vocational adjustment of rural, mildly handicapped students', Exceptional Children 52, pp. 115–121.

Fourqurean, J. M. and T. LaCourt: 1990, 'A follow-up of former special education students: A model for program evaluation', Remedial and Special Education 12, pp. 16–23.

Frank, A. R., P. L. Sitlington, L. Cooper and V. Cool" 1990, 'Adult adjustment of recent graduates of Iowa mental disabilities programs', Education and Training in Mental Retardation 25, pp. 62–75.

Haring, K. A. and D. L. Lovett: 1990, 'A follow-up study of special education graduates', The Journal of Special Education 23, pp. 463–477.

Haring, K. and D. Lovett: 1990, 'A study of the social and vocational adjustment of young adults with mental retardation', Education and Training in Mental Retardation 25, pp. 52–61.

Hasazi, S. B., L. R. Gordon and C. A. Roe: 1985, 'Factors associated with the employment status of handicapped youth exiting high school from 1979 to 1983', Exceptional Children 51, pp. 455–469.

Hasazi, S. B., L. R. Gordon, C. A. Roe, K. Finck, M. Hull and G. Salembier: 1985, 'A statewide follow-up on post high school employment and residential status of students labeled, "mentally retarded"', Education and Training of the Mentally Retarded 20, pp. 222–234.

Hill, M. L., P. H. Wehman, J. Kregel, P. D. Banks and H. M. D. Metzler: 1987, 'Employment outcomes for people with moderate and severe disabilities: an eight-year longitudinal analysis of supported competitive employment', Journal of The Association for Persons with Severe Handicaps 12, pp. 182–189.

Humes, C. H. and G. Brammer: 1985, 'LD career success after high school', Academic Therapy 21, pp. 171–176.

Kortering, L. J. and E. B. Edgar: 1988, 'Vocational rehabilitation and special education: A need for cooperation', Rehabilitation Counselling Bulletin 31, pp. 178–184.

Kregel, J., P. Wehman, J. Seyfarth and K. Marshall: 1986, 'Community integration of young adults with mental retardation: Transition from school to adulthood', Education and Training of the Mentally Retarded 21, pp. 35–42.

Leone, P.: 1984, 'A descriptive follow-up of behaviorally disordered adolescents', Behavioral Disorders 9, pp. 207–214.

Leone, P., R. Fitzmartin, F. Stetson and J. Foster: 1986, 'A retrospective follow-up of behaviorally disordered adolescents: Identifying predictors of treatment outcome', Behavioral Disorders 11, pp. 87–97.

Levine, E. K., N. Zigmond and J. W. Birch: 1985, 'A follow-up study of 52 learning disabled adolescents', Journal of Learning Disabilities 18, pp. 2–7.

Liebert, D., L. Lutsky and A. Gottlieb: 1990, 'Postsecondary experiences of young adults with severe physical disabilities', Exceptional Children 57, pp. 56–63.

McDevitt, S. C., P. M. Smith, D. W. Schmidt and M. Rosen: 1978, 'The deinstitutionalized citizen: Adjustment and quality of life', Mental Retardation 16, pp. 22–24.

Mithaug, D. E., C. N. Horiuchi and P. N. Fanning: 1985, 'A report on the Colorado statewide follow-up survey of special education students', Exceptional Children 51, pp. 397–404.

Neel, R. S., N. Meadows, P. Levine and E. B. Edgar: 1988 'What happens after special education: A statewide follow-up study of secondary students who have behavioral disorders', Behavioral Disorders 13, pp. 209–216.

Neubert, D. A., G. P. Tilson, Jr., and R. N. Ianacone: 1989, 'Postsecondary transition needs and employment patterns of individuals with mild disabilities', Exceptional Children 55, pp. 494–500.

O'Brien, P. J. and W. J. Schiller: 1979, 'Evaluation of a transitional training program for mentally retarded, multiply handicapped high school students', Rehabilitation Literature 40, pp. 232–235.

Pilley, J.: 1988, 'Plans and outcomes: A study of the transition of the Vancouver School Board's 1987 mentally handicapped graduates', B.C. Journal of Special Education 12, pp. 201–213.

Roessler, R. T., D. E. Brolin and J. M. Johnson: 1990, 'Factors affecting employment success and quality of life: A one year follow-up of students in special education', Career Development for Exceptional Individuals 13, pp. 95–107.

Schalock, R., and M. Lilley: 1986, 'Placement from community-based mental retardation programs: How well do clients do 8–10 years later?', American Journal of Mental Deficiency 90, pp. 669–676.

Schalock, R. L., B. Wolzen, I. Ross, B. Elliott, G. Werbel and K. Peterson: 1986, 'Post-secondary community placement of handicapped students: A five-year follow-up', Learning disability Quarterly 9, pp. 295–303.

Scuccimarra, D. J. and D. L. Speece: 1990, 'Employment outcomes and social integration of students with mild handicaps: The quality of life two years after high school', Journal of Learning Disabilities 23, pp. 213–219.

Sitlington, P. L. and A. R. Frank: 1990, 'Are adolescents with learning disabilities successfully crossing the bridge into adult life', Learning disabilities quarterly 13, pp. 97–111.

Valdes, K. A., C. L. Williamson and M. M. Wagner: 1990, The National Longitudinal Transition Study of Special Education Students (SRI International, Menlo Park, CA).

Wehman, P., M. Hill, P. Goodall, P. Cleveland, V. Brooke and J. H. Pentecost, Jr.: 1982, 'Job placement and follow-up of moderately and severely handicapped individuals after three years', Journal of the Association for Persons with Severe Handicaps 7, pp. 5–16.

Wehman, P., C. Jasper, W. Parent, S. Miller, W. Wood, J. Marchant, C. M. Talbert and R. Walker: 1989, 'From school to competitive employment for young adults with mental retardation: Transition in practice', Career Development for Exceptional Individuals 12, pp. 97–105.

Wehman, P., J. Kregel and J. Seyfarth: 1985, 'Employment outlook for young adults with mental retardation', Rehabilitation Counselling Bulletin 29, pp. 90–99.

Wehman, P., J. Kregel and J. Seyfarth: 1985, 'Transition from school to work for individuals with severe handicaps: A follow-up study', Journal of the Association for Persons with Severe Handicaps 10, pp. 132–136.

White, W. J., G. R. Alley, D. D. Deshler, J. B. Schumaker, M. M. Warner and F. L. Clark: 1982, 'Are there learning disabilities after high school?', Exceptional Children 49, pp. 273–274.

Zetlin, A. G. and A. Hosseini: 1989, 'Six postschool case studies of mildly learning handicapped young adults', Exceptional Children 55, pp. 405–411.
Zigmond, N. and H. Thornton: 1985, 'Follow-up of postsecondary age learning disabled graduates and drop-outs', Learning Disabilities research 1, pp. 50–55.

University of Oregon,
Department of Education,
College of Education,
Eugene OR 97403–1211,
U.S.A.

DAVID M. ROMNEY, ROY I. BROWN AND PREM S. FRY

IMPROVING THE QUALITY OF LIFE:
PRESCRIPTIONS FOR CHANGE

(Accepted 14 February, 1994)

ABSTRACT. The main points made in the previous papers are summarized and integrated and the strategies that the authors have recommended for producing an improved QOL are discussed. QOL is also systematically reviewed in relation to matters of definition, assessment, applications, and directions for future research and practice.

The main thrust of this special issue has been to consider policies and practices for improving the quality of life (QOL) of people in general and, especially, of those individuals who are afflicted with a mental or physical disability. This disability might arise at conception or during childhood or manifest itself for the first time in old age; it might be a chronic mental disorder such as schizophrenia or a chronic deteriorating physical illness such as AIDS. Regardless of the nature of the disability, the effects on a person's QOL can be devastating. What steps, therefore, should be taken to counter these effects? Is it possible for individuals who are disabled to enjoy a QOL comparable to that typically enjoyed by people who are not disabled?

The term "disability" is fully defined in the *International Classification of Impairments, Disabilities and Handicaps* (WHO, 1980) where the distinction between "impairment," "disability" and "handicap" is made clear. *Impairment* is defined as "any loss or abnormality of psychological, physiological or anatomical structure or function." *Disability* is defined as "any restriction or lack (resulting from an impairment) of ability to perform an activity in a manner or within the range considered normal for a human being." *Handicap* is defined as "a disadvantage for an individual, resulting from an impairment or disability, that prevents or limits the fulfilment of a role that is normal (depending on age, sex, and social and cultural factors) for that individual." Consequently, disability in the ideal environment does not have to be a handicap. This is the challenge for QOL as its proponents seek to lessen handicap and reduce dependency. It is, therefore, closely connected with the modification of the environment, which includes people's negative stereotypes. Thus, QOL has psychological as well as sociological and economic connotations.

We are concerned not only with individuals who are disabled but with *all* individuals, particularly those who are experiencing major stress. How can *their* QOL be improved? The specific recommendations that have been made by the various authors who have contributed papers to this issue may seem at first glance to be as different as the target populations themselves. Yet closer inspection reveals a common thread which binds them together and gives them wider currency. In this concluding paper these are some of the issues we will be addressing; other issues relate more to methodology.

We realize that we may have at least two audiences: the scientists who are preoccupied with methodological issues such as research design, assessment tools, and outcome measures in QOL studies, and the professionals, practitioners, economists and politicians who are more interested in how the findings from scientific studies translate into achieving solid social policy relevance. While we hope to be able to satisfy the interests of both audiences, we take this opportunity to remind our readers that the primary focus of this book has to do with *improving* QOL rather than with advancing theory. We hope, incidentally, that there is a third audience of concerned citizens, ombudsmen, and humanists who will appreciate both the scientific and the practical aspects of the topic and will act as advocates for people with disabilities in their struggle to enhance their QOL.

RECOMMENDATIONS

Aside from Trevor Parmenter, who dealt with conceptual and measurement issues, all the contributors have made some recommendations for making tangible improvements to QOL. With respect to QOL in the general population, David Evans calls for more research to identify the relative importance of those factors appearing to contribute to QOL and the best way to measure them. He also argues in favour of longitudinal outcome studies to evaluate the relative efficacy of programs designed to improve QOL before committing funds to any particular approach. He is consequently somewhat tentative about making specific recommendations. Nevertheless, he stresses the importance of *education* at all age levels, starting at kindergarten and continuing throughout adulthood, to help individuals adopt a healthier life style and acquire essential coping skills. Here the media could have a useful role to play in promoting suitable programs. For those individuals who are at risk for a diminished QOL, social support groups should be established. With regard to modifying the environment to enhance QOL, programs directed towards this end could be facilitated by legislation (Stokols, 1992).

Marcia Ory and Donna Cox make substantive recommendations for enhancing the QOL of elderly individuals. First and foremost, to offset the frailty that often accompanies old age, they emphasize the importance of a healthy lifestyle (i.e., regular exercise, a sensible diet, and the avoidance of risk factors such as smoking and excessive drinking). Regular exercise, in particular, such as brisk walking, is seen as indispensable. In addition, because older persons tend to dismiss aches and pains, insomnia, incontinence and other complaints as a natural part of aging, they may have to be encouraged to seek medical advice (for prevention as well as intervention). This is a good example of how QOL is dependent on the perceptions of both the client and the professional.

Besides physical infirmities, a common problem associated with old age which diminishes QOL is *loneliness* resulting from social isolation, a problem that is sometimes compounded by sensory isolation such as deafness. For this reason social support and social networking become paramount. It has been shown conclusively that mortality is delayed for individuals with active social lives (Berkman and Breslow, 1989) whereas the loss or absence of familiar sources of social support have been linked to heart disease, accidents, suicides, commitments to mental hospital, truancy, ulcers, cancer, and schizophrenia (Bruhn and Philips,

1984). In other words, social activity would appear to advance both *quantity* and *quality* of life.

To encourage the development of better QOL it will be necessary for change of occur in many social institutions. For instance, as people get older they may go out less often at night. Because of diminishing stamina and poorer dark adaptation, seniors tend to do their community activities during daylight. This has major implications for the opening hours of theatres, restaurants, shopping malls, etc. It also has implications for such things as theatre lighting and program print size (Brown, 1993). The implications of an aging population for environmental changes are therefore wide-ranging. Having recreational and cultural facilities open when elderly people are able to visit them is important for developing and maintaining friendship and support networks. As we know, social isolation is one of the principal challenges facing older widowed women.

The identification of QOL with health status culminates in the paper by Bob Kaplan. Here the two concepts are virtually synonymous and QOL is expressed in terms of QALYs. Kaplan argues that "available resources be used to produce the greatest benefit for the greatest number of people". He is most concerned about the *cost-effectiveness* of existing health programs and has devised an elaborate algorithm for computing a "utility" ratio to determine whether a given procedure is worthwhile. Using such diverse examples as seat-belt legislation as a way to lessen injury and the tobacco tax as a way to reduce the consumption of cigarettes, he illustrates that an ounce of prevention is better than a pound of cure. On the other hand, he demonstrates that the evidence in favour of the value of neonatal circumcision for preventing penile cancer and urinary tract infections is less convincing. In this paper, with much ingenuity, Kaplan shows us how we can combine measurement studies with policy analysis.

Although we of course agree that good health is an important ingredient of QOL, and notwithstanding the legitimacy of Kaplan's approach, we question whether health status is or should be the be-all and end-all. For many authorities QOL encompasses more than the state of one's health. The novelist and playwright John Mortimer's best known fictional character, the barrister Horace Rumpole, once complained bitterly how his quality of life had deteriorated since his doctor placed him on a meagre, low cholesterol diet! And Mortimer, himself, objects to governmental legislation curtailing his freedom to smoke. The point is that *life satisfaction*, another important ingredient of QOL, does not enter into Kaplan's formula. In other words, the subjective element of QOL is missing. The fact remains that relief of symptoms does not inevitably result in an elevated QOL, nor do their exacerbation necessarily lower QOL. How the individual *reacts* to the illness is, at least to some degree, separate from the illness itself.

In contrast to Kaplan, Céline Mercier stresses the importance of subjective factors in determining QOL, pointing out that there are often discrepancies between them and objective factors. In her consideration of individuals with chronic mental disorders, she draws attention to how they *personally perceive* their abilities to carry out daily activities and fulfil roles. If these perceptions are positive, they are more likely to be satisfied with their lives and to remain in the community, as opposed to re-entering an institution. The implications for programs designed to improve QOL are that they should always include interventions for *personal growth* and for boosting *self-efficacy* and *self-esteem* as well as for raising overall level of functioning by improving coping skills and problem-solving abilities. This should result in greater life satisfaction and emotional well-being. However, because life satisfaction is based on how one's perceptions of one's own situation compared with one's expectations – the so-called Gap Principle (Calman, 1984) – people in similar circumstances but with different expectations would have different levels of QOL, with the person with the higher expectations having the lower QOL.

QOL seems to be viewed rather differently in different professional spheres. Not only do definitions differ, but so do the underlying concepts. These differences lead to various and diverse models and applications. In the (biological) health field, QOL tends to be interpreted as a physical phenomenon which should be measured objectively. In the mental health field and the field of disability it is viewed more multidimensionally with both subjective and objective elements. In some studies (e.g., Bateson, 1972; Campbell, 1981; Zautra and Reich, 1983) subjective measures have played the dominant role. However, if we believe that QOL is an entirely subjective experience, it would follow that one could boost QOL merely by lowering one's expectations, a line of reasoning which runs clearly counter to the general understanding of what is meant by QOL. Nevertheless, raising an individual's awareness of his or her *potential* could contribute to a higher QOL provided this awareness spurs the individual to appropriate action.

In making her recommendations for improving QOL, Mercier does not neglect the objective determinants of QOL. She is aware of the traditional indicators of QOL such as health, employment and leisure, social relations and finances. Improvement of living conditions is often a top priority for individuals who are mentally unstable since they usually have little control over their environment. In fact, their mental disorder makes them especially vulnerable to exploitation and victimization. It is clear that there is a need to "sensitize" the community to this problem so that at the very least it will ensure the safety and protect the rights of people with mental disorders. But communities must also remember that people who have a mental illness are like the rest of us inasmuch as they also have a desire for intimacy, romance, and matrimony and that our responsibility does not end there. The lack of friends and partners for people who have a mental illness (or a develop- mental disability) aggravates the difficulties these people have in leading normal lifestyles. To overcome their isolation, more attention needs to be paid by professionals to solving the problem of social networking. Indeed the lack of normal friendships and social networks constitute two of the most challenging handicaps for people with mental illness or developmental disability (Denholm, 1993; Firth and Rapley, 1990). Yet the importance of these aspects of QOL tends to be minimized by researchers and practitioners working with these populations. This has serious implications for how research is devised and how concepts of QOL are implemented.

Finally, we turn to the paper by Andy Halpern on adolescents with developmental disabilities who are experiencing the transition from school to the workplace. What does he recommend to improve the QOL of these individuals? Halpern discusses the different types of school-based programs that have been implemented to facilitate this transition and finds them wanting. The goals of the programs have tended to focus on employment at the expense of other aspects of QOL. He recommends that a more comprehensive approach to outcomes is needed which would include physical and mental well-being, performance of valued adult roles, and self-fulfilment. These goals closely resemble those advocated by Mercier in the preceding paper. Instead of being limited to vocational instruction, school-based and community programs should employ a variety of techniques that will enable all the other aspects of QOL to be achieved. Furthermore, because the average young person is far from being a passive recipient of external influences, but is an active agent who brings a set of attitudes, values, dispositions and motivations to bear on his or her experiences, we concur with Halpern that adolescents with disabilities should be set upon the path of self-determination by being given encouragement to exert control over their own transition experiences which play such a critical role in shaping adult identity.

The concept of transition periods is seen as important within the field of special education, and Halpern underlines some of the steps that need to be taken to move from school to the adult world. But there are many transition points throughout life and educational experiences are increasingly being designed to cope with them (e.g., counselling schemes to prepare for retirement). However, maintenance or improvement of QOL is frequently not taken into account when planning these experiences. The issue of transition raises, almost paradoxically, the importance of treating QOL as a *life-span issue*, for individuals face transitions at various ages and these often represent periods of stress (cf. Erikson, 1968; Marcia, 1966). Sometimes they are life-threatening and almost always are associated with QOL. And even when they are not life-threatening, "there may be critical periods of exposure to risk which influence health and functioning outcomes"; these are referred to by Ory and Cox "windows of vulnerability". The life-span approach to QOL, therefore, has relevance for any model of QOL and becomes central to its definition.

Some models concerned with enhancing the QOL of the general population are concerned essentially with developing interventions to improve the functional independence of individuals on all rungs of the developmental ladder. But the fact remains that the reviews of scientific studies presented in the various papers in this volume and the generic models proposed, place an uncommon emphasis on attributes of the subjects and respondents that are time-based and process-related. Most undertake to answer questions concerning demographic variations and temporal variations in QOL assessments and standards required to assess outcomes. Although studies of time-related variables are immensely useful in studying the dynamics of change at single points of time, nonetheless, all these studies must be conceptualized as base-line studies against which changes in the future should be assessed. Inferences drawn from these studies, especially for the purposes of policy relevance of these materials, or for purposes of scientific understanding of human growth or deterioration with aging, must remain severely constrained without true longitudinal data collected over a reasonable span of time.

THE COMMON THREAD

Inspection of the various recommendations made by the contributors for improving QOL suggests that the goals are essentially similar and that differences are due to the degree of emphasis they receive. Moreover, these differences in emphasis are not arbitrary but appear to reflect the nature of the disabilities associated with the disabled population being considered. Thus for individuals with health problems, i.e., the chronically sick and the frail elderly, health promotion is paramount. Whereas for people with mental disorders and developmental disabilities, psychological factors such as well-being and self-worth assume greater prominence. It would seem, therefore, that the objective/subjective QOL dichotomy is manifested to a certain extent among *all* the different populations. But this dichotomy is far from absolute: for people with health problems the importance of social networking has already been mentioned; and for people with mental disorders or developmental disabilities, material conditions and employment are objective factors that loom large in determining the quality of their lives.

Although Evans did make specific recommendations on how to improve QOL in the general population, he hesitated to do so because he believes we lack the knowledge on which to base our judgments;

however, other contributors give examples of successful interventions with individuals who are disabled. Ory and Cox note that intensive educational efforts and advertising campaigns have been effective in promoting behaviours which prevent or alleviate chronic health problems of older people living in the community and that customized programs or environments (e.g., Special Care Units) hold promise for those individuals residing in institutions.

For Mercier, the hallmark of QOL is independent living and she argues forcefully that adequate social and behavioural services should be provided to enable (former) psychiatric patients to live independently in the community. These services include programs directed at daily living activities such as self-care, managing finances, interpersonal relations, and planning for the future. Moreover, the importance of hobbies and other leisure activities for QOL should not be neglected. Of course Mercier realizes that the degree of autonomy possible is related to functional level, and the goal of independent living may not be feasible for individuals whose disorder is so severe that they can only function at a very low level. These individuals will require some sort of residential care, depending on the extent of their impairment, ranging from an institution (most restrictive) though group home, foster/parental home, and sheltered accommodation, to independent living situations (least restrictive). As mentioned previously, how these individuals *perceive* their environment and their personal aspirations must be taken into account when assessing and attempting to change their QOL. Individual programming and counselling, therefore, become desirable.

In general, the recommendations made by Mercier for improving the QOL of adults with psychiatric disorders also apply to adults with developmental disabilities (Schalock, 1990). Halpern, however, deals in his paper with adolescents who are on the verge of leaving school. But the question of independent living is as pressing an issue for this population as any other. Like all older adolescents, those challenged by developmental disabilities are typically concerned about their employment prospects; and the resolution of this concern lies at the heart of Halpern's paper. Again, he warns us not to overlook the importance of subjective factors in evaluating QOL. The program he describes involves a network of community transition teams which focus on program development in order to provide students with disabilities with appropriate vocational instruction to prepare them for jobs in their communities. The program succeeded in its immediate aims and, amongst the indirect benefits, a "tremendous esprit de corps emerged, accompanied by a growing sense of self-worth and self-esteem." There seems little doubt that the QOL of the participants spontaneously improved as a result of the successful outcome. However, in other studies (e.g., Brown *et al.*, 1992) employment has not been found to be the key issue in rehabilitation. Emotional and recreational needs, particularly in relation to the family, are often identified as more important by consumers and family sponsors. This is especially true in the case of individuals with severe physical and/or mental disabilities resulting from congenital defects or traumatic injuries later in life.

DEFINITION

The fact that QOL is such an elusive concept has resulted in countless attempts to define it. Because of the difficulty in specifying the term, no universally accepted definition is available. There are several reasons for this. First is the fact that psychological processes relevant to experiences of QOL can be described and interpreted through many different conceptual filters and languages. Discrepancies between the views of different writers may occur in the basic contents of the models they present, the facts they address, and the features they describe and whether their models are "top-down" or "bottom-up." It is thus rarely possible to integrate the models of QOL proposed by different authors (Warr, 1987).

A second difficulty in reaching a consensus about how QOL should be defined and promoted arises from the fact that the concept of QOL is to a considerable degree *value-laden*; several authors and researchers seek to map descriptive statements on to an evaluation dimension. Processes and outcomes which are designated as "superior" QOL are typically those accepted and valued by contemporary society, *often by the middle class of that society.*

A third difficulty in reaching general agreement about a definition of QOL arises from the fact that the concept embodies the understanding of human growth and developmental processes, the average life-span of individuals within their communities, and the extent to which these psychological processes are influenced by environmental factors and individual value systems. The "uniformity myth" that implies that all individuals, regardless of age and class, are similarly affected needs to be seriously challenged.

Although both subjective and objective factors are important in determining QOL, three of our contributors – Halpern, Mercier, and Parmenter – seem to favour the subjective perspective, whereas two of them – Evans and Kaplan – lean more towards objective criteria. Granted that subjective indicators may have lower measurement reliability than objective indicators, if we accept the proposition that QOL can only be judged in the last resort by the individuals themselves on the basis of their own idiosyncratic needs and standards, subjective factors would still remain the preferred kind of indicator. It seems to us, therefore, that the *ultimate* determinant of QOL is psychological well-being. This does not mean that QOL is synonymous with perceived QOL, but it does mean we need to assess the substantive interpretations that individuals place upon its environmental determinants.

Both Halpern and Evans have produced "taxonomies" of QOL, i.e., classifications of its main features, which they discuss in their respective papers. Using structural equation modelling, Romney *et al.* (1992) confirmed the presence of five major components in cardiac patients: symptoms of illness, illness-related deficit, interpersonal relationships, morale, and economic-employment circumstances. The five same factors were found to apply in a study of schizophrenic patients (Romney, 1994), suggesting that they may be the key QOL factors for people with physical and mental illnesses. It is noteworthy that Kaplan focuses on only the first two of these five factors in his paper.

MEASUREMENT MODELS

Because there is a growing consensus that QOL is multidimensional, there is less enthusiasm these days for utilizing a global index. To quote Parmenter: "Rather than attempting to use a single index as a measure of quality of life, it would seem more reasonable to ask the question for what purpose will the data be. used and to design an instrument that does not purport to come up with a single score." Other authors besides Parmenter (e.g., Brown *et al.*, 1992; Cummins, 1992; Schalock, 1991) have commented on the *holistic* nature of QOL extending, as it does, through such varied domains as wellness, social networks, employment, home and family living, social skills, and leisure and recreation, and encompassing the total life-span. In fact, there seems to be a remarkable degree of agreement on this point, at least among researchers in the field of developmental disability (Felce and Perry, 1993).

Most, if not all, agree on the significance of *social perception* in determining disability and handicap and in this and other contexts emphasize the importance of subjective factors such as choice, empowerment, and self-image. These factors seem to play a lesser role in the health literature on QOL though recent studies on cancer, for instance, have begun to take these factors into account (e.g., Osaba, 1991; Schipper *et al.*, 1984). Parmenter is critical of the use of QALYs because they aggregate the quality and quantity of survival into a single variable. He also challenges the assumptions on which QALYs are based, namely, that the same algorithm should apply to all people suffering from a particular disease irrespective of age (with which QOL correlates positively), and that the quality versus quantity decisions are not usually made by the people suffering from the disease. Whether one emphasizes objective or subjective data, because individuals weight the importance of the various aspects of QOL differently, the person whose life quality is being assessed must be allowed to participate in the process if the results of the assessment are to be credible. Furthermore, the selection of items to be included in the assessment instrument should be influenced by the views of the population under study. Recognition of the importance of the consumer's perspective is evident in the titles of several articles focusing on psychiatric patients (McIntyre *et al.*, 1989;

Pinkney *et al.*, 1991; Thapa *et al.*, 1989), and variability of perceptions and needs amongst individuals with disabilities is one of the principal characteristics of QOL studies. Thus, Ory and Cox give a specific example of how the helping professional and the older woman may have different interpretations of what is meant by "treatment success." "Is the intervention only a success," they ask, "if the subjects remain dry, or does success constitute some measure of improvement in incontinence?" Because individuals differ in their preferences, a woman with a major incontinence problem may be satisfied with a reduced number of episodes, whereas those with more active lifestyles may want more assurance.

Finally, in addition to psychometric properties such as face and content validity and reliability, what is most needed – and here we concur with Parmenter – are construct validation studies. One has to demonstrate empirically a "nomological network" of laws expressing the functional properties of QOL in relation to other (psychosocial and biological) constructs and the observations used to measure them.

STRUCTURAL MODELS

We need to be able to place QOL on a firm theoretical footing because theory can act as a guide and impetus for further research and provide a sound rationale for assessment and intervention. In turning to our contributors we find that several of our authors – Evans, Ory and Cox, and Halpern – offer explicit structural models of QOL. According to Evans, QOL may be construed as the ultimate outcome variable in a four-stage model (see Figure 1 in his paper). Personality and environmental factors (stage 1) act on general and specific skills, positive and negative emotion, and social support (stage 2) which in turn influence the cognitive appraisal of life circumstances (stage 3) which determines, and is determined by, QOL (stage 4). Change to any one or more of these preceding factors could affect QOL, for better or worse. In the Ory and Cox model, QOL is also designated as an outcome measure, but just one of several indicators of health or illness. It is seen as a function of aging, the sociocultural environment, and health attitudes and behaviours as well as psychosocial and biological mechanisms, which in turn it can influence (see Figure 2 in their paper). While this model is perhaps too general to be of practical use, it elucidates the dynamic nature of the aging process on QOL. Halpern's model, which is depicted in Figure 2 in his paper, suggests that QOL can be influenced by student and family characteristics, school services, and school achievement. He distinguishes in his model between QOL in school and QOL out of school and assumes that the latter is affected by the former (but not the other way round). Also, QOL outside school affects, and is affected by, post-school services. From this model we can infer that QOL can be enhanced by changing one or more of the causative factors; for instance, a rise in school achievement should, according this model, enhance QOL.

Unlike the Ory and Cox's "saturated" model, with reciprocal pathways going everywhere, both Halpern's and Evans' models could be tested statistically by means of covariance-structure analysis (also known as structural equation modelling or SEM for short) using computer programs such as LISREL or EQS to ascertain how well it fits actual data. A good fit would imply that the model may be correct and that it would be worthwhile testing experimentally. The significance of this kind of analysis was recognized almost a decade ago by Ware (1984) who predicted "we will soon see attempts to estimate the structure of the various components of health status, including their relationships at a point in time and their interdependencies over time (p. 2317)."

Covariance-structure analysis was first used in QOL research by Andrews and Withey (1976) who viewed the experience of general well-being as the product of personal characteristics, objective life conditions in various domains, and satisfaction with life conditions in these various domains. Their model of QOL subsequently served as the basis for the construction of one of the first scales (Lehman, 1983) to assess the QOL of psychiatric patients, a scale used by Mercier in a SEM study designed to investigate how autonomy and service utilization could influence the QOL and community tenure of psychotic patients (Mercier and King, in press). Halpern *et al.* (1986) tested a causal model of quality of life showing the functional relationships between client satisfaction, occupation, residential environment and social support/

safety in a sample of adults with mental retardation. LISREL was also used ingeniously by Lance *et al.* (1989) to compare "top-down", "bottom-up", and "bidirectional" models of QOL on a sample of academics (see paper by Evans), and also by Romney *et al.* (1992) in an attempt to decide whether the physical and mental symptoms exhibited by cardiac patients could be held responsible for lowering the psychosocial components of quality of life or, conversely, whether psychosocial factors could be to blame for aggravating the symptoms. These are just a few, varied examples of the application of covariance-structure analysis to exploring and confirming conceptual models of QOL that might have consequences for both assessment and intervention strategies.

A HIERARCHY OF NEEDS

Theories of QOL tend to be self-contained. Can they be brought within a broader framework of social psychological theory? If so, what would be the implications for improving QOL in disabled and nondisabled populations? The potential value of the answers to these questions merits further discussion. In the context of the life-span approach to QOL, the importance of personal goals is magnified and that is why some QOL researchers have leaned heavily on the theoretical formulation of Maslow (1968) who has tried to explain human motivation in terms of a hierarchy of needs (usually represented pictorially by a pyramid). These needs have to be satisfied (at least partially) in a certain order beginning with physiological needs essential for survival such as hunger, thirst and sex at the base of the pyramid and ending with the need for self-actualization or the realization of one's potential at the apex. Between these two extremes lie (in ascending order) the need for safety, the need for affection and acceptance, and the need for respect and self-esteem. When people lose their jobs because of mandatory retirement or because a serious mental or physical illness supervenes, their income diminishes and, as a result, they often experience a "needs shift" (Borgen and Amundson, 1984). Their needs fall down the hierarchy and they find themselves seeking to fulfil needs at a much lower level. They are now obliged to attend to needs which had erstwhile been taken for granted. For example, a threat to material insecurity will prompt them to start worrying about meeting physical safety and comfort needs.

Even amongst those people in the general population who do not feel threatened by financial insecurity, total self-actualization is seldom achieved. Many elderly people often feel neglected and unwanted and those who are infirm and cannot manage very well on their own may have reduced self-esteem. This may also be true of people with chronic physical disorders who cannot fend for themselves and have to rely heavily on others. This is why it is so important to enable them to live as autonomously as possible.

For those individuals with chronic mental disorders who are discharged from institutions and are not adequately supported by social services in the community, the picture is even more grim. They often find themselves in dire straits as "street people" whose basic biological needs for food and shelter are not met. Their needs start at the bottom level of Maslow's hierarchy. Those who live in sheltered accommodation may have their basic needs fulfilled but they may still be vulnerable to abuse and exploitation. And even those who are physically safe, still crave acceptance, affection and respect.

What applies to individuals with chronic mental disorders also applies, as Halpern points out, to adolescents with developmental disabilities. For them employment opportunities are not enough: if they do not have the "power" to make their own choices and to strive for their own goals, they will realize that other people decide things for them and their self-esteem will suffer. Without a sense of self-worth, they will tend to view themselves in a negative fashion and perceive the world similarly. On the other hand, if they see themselves as instrumental in accomplishing their personal goals (self-efficacy), this will be manifested in confidence about their ability to change the course of events in other spheres of life and is generally accompanied by a sense of "internal" as opposed to "external" locus of control (Rotter, 1966).

Although the pyramid of needs may apply to most people in most circumstances, there are always exceptions. Halpern gives an example from Edgerton (1990) of a person who felt self-actualized despite (or maybe because of) living in a dangerous environment and having unhealthy relationships. Sometimes individuals have the ability to transcend the needs and aspirations of ordinary people and live saintly and self-fulfilling lives. Again this example reminds us of the importance of the subjective perspective in evaluating QOL. What society may consider to be a low level of QOL may be viewed by the individual concerned as just the opposite.

NORMALIZATION AND THE POWER TO CHOOSE

Although it is apparent that the study of quality of life has taken different routes for differently disabled populations, there is nevertheless considerable overlap among the various areas. The movement to discharge people from custodial institutions in the Western World was closely tied to the emergence of the "normalization movement" which has recognized the importance of the development of normal lifestyles for each individual within the setting of a natural environment. In an attempt to clarify what is meant by "normalization", Wolfensberger (1987) renamed it *social role valorization*. In order to be valued, people have to be seen to be carrying out valued tasks. Moreover, QOL depends not only on the value placed upon these activities (or what one wears or where one lives) by the individual, but also on how they are valued by other people in the community, especially those professionals who come into contact with the individuals concerned. As it is the professionals who decide who receives treatment, and so on, the issue of quality of life becomes an issue of their professional philosophy and ethical practice. This has important implications for both policy making and educational planning.

Crucial to any QOL model consistent with the aims of this movement is a recognition that, wherever possible, individuals should be able to choose the interventions they prefer within natural environments, rather than institutions such as rehabilitation centres, hospitals of schools. This means relying much more on the perceptions of the individuals concerned. For those individuals who cannot express themselves because they suffer from a cognitive impairment (dysphasia) or articulatory impairment (dysarthria), attempts have been made to assess perception of QOL by nonverbal means. Results suggest that even very disabled persons are capable of making choices that are meaningful and realistic (Autio, 1992; Cummins, 1992).

Nowhere perhaps does the issue of choice become more apparent, and Mercier has drawn our attention to this finding, than in the realm of leisure and recreation. Many people with disabilities tend to assume the spectator role, which reinforces their marginalization and feelings of disempowerment. Social and physical recreational activities tend to build self-image, increase motivation, and often improve fitness and health. It is possible for these reasons that individuals with physical handicaps who obtain re-employment are frequently those who are very active in their leisure and recreation time. Although normative data are inadequate, there is some evidence of a poor balance of activity within various disabled populations compared with the normal population.

Other authors have stressed the relevance of recreation and leisure for people with physical disabilities (Day, 1989) and developmental handicaps (Emes and Ferris, 1986) as a means of promoting wellness, strengthening social networks and obtaining employment. Unfortunately, because our society is so work-oriented, "leisure and recreation" are regarded as frivolous activities by governments which tend to look askance at requests for funding of research and implementation of programs in these areas. Their development, however, seems critical for any broad model of QOL. Recreation and leisure, we believe, should be set in the context of normalization. This would nicely identify the complex nature of QOL since both the activities and the environment in which they take place are important considerations. It does not follow of course that when it comes to competitive sports, people who are disabled would prefer to compete against people who are not. As Halpern has noted, there are segregated competitions, e.g., Special Olympics, dedicated to individuals with physical handicaps. The point is that they have the opportunity to compete at all, thereby putting them on a par with the rest of humanity. In keeping with the principle of freedom of choice, people with disabilities should have the right to decide for themselves whether they wish to indulge in integrated recreational activities are not.

Granted that freedom of choice is of such importance, it is surprising that in measuring QOL, cultural differences are often ignored. To people of different cultures, whether living in their homelands or as new immigrants to the West, QOL may have an entirely different meaning from our own. The cultural relativity of the quality of life concept has been investigated by Hofstede (1984) who commented: "Researchers approaching the issue in Third World countries have relied too much on definitions of 'quality' derived from North American and ... West European values" (p. 397). He found that cultural differences could be explained largely in terms of four dimensions: power distance, which is the extent to which the less powerful person in society accepts inequality in power and considers it normal; individualism as opposed to collectivism; masculinity as opposed to femininity, i.e., the opposition of social roles; uncertainty avoidance, which defines the extent to which people tolerate uncertainty and ambiguity and the extent they try to avoid such situations by being dogmatic. Hofstede plotted 50 countries and three regions on these dimensions, thereby determining their relative importance to each country. For example: "In Southeast Asian cultures, preserving harmony with one's social environment [i.e., collectivism] is a powerful motivator. People would probably define high quality of life as one in which harmony is achieved and preserved" (p. 394). Thus Maslow's hierarchy of needs, where the emphasis is on autonomy and individualism, with self-actualization as the highest goal, may be regarded as *ethnocentric*. Different cultures would appear to have different needs hierarchies and there is no justification for imposing Western values on them all.

Because the assumptions that govern QOL in one culture may not hold for another, this does not imply that we should abandon the objective of comparing QOL data across cultures. However, the psychometric properties and meaning of the instrument must be determined in the culture where it is applied for we cannot take it for granted that an instrument is reliable and valid in all cultures and that the same question (and answer) is equivalent in different cultures. Not only is there a need for cross-cultural investigations in foreign countries, but even in the same country where there may be many groups with widely differing ethnic backgrounds, cultural factors must be taken into account when assessing their QOL. It is noteworthy that according to Ory and Cox the United States National Institute on Aging has recently been focusing research attention on ethnic minorities. This is heartening news; however, a timely reminder from Sartorius (1987) that knowledge about and involvement with other cultures has a more important function than understanding and assessment "makes us remember the larger family of man and the obligation to learn to help others, regardless of their looks and addresses, their races, size, and language" (p. 23). We cannot escape the fact that QOL is a *universal obligation*.

COST-EFFECTIVENESS

QOL models which are cost-effective are likely to be very attractive to governments. Consequently, utilitarian approaches to QOL such as the one put forward by Kaplan, which stress the economic impact of disease, would tend to receive governmental approval. From the point of view of the consumer who is disabled and professionals working in the field, it is also politically expedient to "sell" QOL models to the public on the grounds that savings can be made from such developments. Many of the goals of the normalization QOL movement lend themselves to cost-effective implementation for various types of health interventions, e.g., the possibility of using local day clinics rather than hospital beds. However, costs are not always reduced. For instance, when people who are mentally ill or developmentally disabled enhance their QOL by living in the community, they often require more support from social services. Similarly, improved QOL for people who are elderly can result in greater longevity with additional attendant costs. Indeed, if one were cynical, one might argue that the most cost-effective measure is death because prolonging life entails costs. It is not a question, therefore, of how much it costs but rather how funds should be distributed.

The issue in our view cannot be resolved in terms of cost savings but must be perceived in terms of empowerment which, of course, is a major criterion of QOL. This position is often misunderstood because people interpret empowerment as a provision of services when in reality it is solely a provision of environments where individuals may come to empower themselves.

COMMUNITY SUPPORT

Although the key to QOL may not lie in the quality and quantity of the social services provided but in adapting the environment to allow the individual who is disabled to live normally, there is undoubtedly still a need for community support. The importance of community support is recognized in several of the papers. In this context the development of advocacy movements, self-help groups, and "brokerage" becomes critical. But there are more specific ways in which the community can be involved. As Mercier mentions in her paper, the literature shows that case management seems to be an effective way of improving the QOL of patients with chronic psychiatric disorders. On the other hand, working in the artificial environment of a sheltered workshop is viewed by these patients as futile, and the activities are referred to scathingly by some of them, according to Mercier, as "Mickey Mouse jobs". Only programs that can facilitate life in the community are truly appreciated. Thus the role of families, neighbours, and volunteer helpers is indispensable. The immediate help they can dispense is threefold: instrumental (i.e., providing materials or services), emotional (i.e., conveying a feeling of caring, love, sympathy, reassurance, belonging, or encouragement), and informational (i.e., giving facts, opinions, advice, feedback, suggestions about reconstruing circumstances or what to do). We concur wholeheartedly with Mercier's conclusion that "intervention strategies should also be developed to help communities become 'competent communities' for their members-in-need." The notion of "competence" in describing a community in this context is particularly apt because too little support can make a person feel helpless, but too much can make people dependent and limit their creativity.

INDIVIDUAL VARIABILITY

In future research on QOL, the "uniformity myth" needs to be dispelled. Much of the work done to date seems to be founded upon the static perspective in which it is assumed that the impact of disabilities and even environmental factors, such as the presence of social support and the availability of control, are constant over the course of the disability. There is now evidence (e.g., Rowland, 1989) showing obvious age and gender differences in the psychosocial impact of disabilities and adaptive demands on QOL across the developmental milestones of adolescence, middle and later adulthood. Similarly, there is evidence (Felton and Revenson, 1987) that various forms of ill health (e.g., diabetes, cancer and arthritis) affect the QOL of individuals differentially at different stages of the life span. These findings provide a stimulating challenge to the uniformity assumptions about the clinical management of individuals at different stages of transition and their expectations about QOL in the immediate and foreseeable future. Practical recommendations for improving QOL must therefore take into account the possible causes of adverse effects on QOL for individuals at different development stages.

The issue of individual variability is often neglected by many writers working in the field of QOL. Although it is important to know how populations respond to interventions based on community models, it is equally important to know how individuals within these populations will respond. To cite Parmenter again: "Quality of life research has overly concentrated on overall changes within groups of patients and has obscured the significance of individual variation." In other words: What do they as individuals feel is important in their life quality? What are the particular challenges they and their families face?

The whole value of normative studies is thus open to question. By labelling individuals through the use of various diagnostic techniques, there is always the danger of *stereotyping* them so that they will be viewed as identical, when in fact there is considerable evidence to the contrary. Ory and Cox bring this point out very clearly when they discuss variability in the aging process. But this is typical of all groups and, in making their point, they are illustrating the trap we have fallen into by labelling people and seeing them as similar. It is evident that any research paradigm must take into account the wide range of variability that occurs. Unfortunately, it is customary just to inspect mean differences in scores across occasions and treatments and to treat the variability of responses that occur in such studies as mere "error variance."

Because QOL models should be founded on issues of individual differences and choices, the desirability of assessing personal perceptions and subjective reality is heightened. In recent years it has become much more common to collect individual life stories and anecdotal accounts before embarking on a full-scale (quantitative) project. Yet research tradition and the preferences of policy-makers require that objective as well as subjective data be amassed. Because of this the arguments of Evans in relation to collecting normative data carry more weight. However, if perceived QOL evaluations are worth pursuing, substantial benefits can be gained by using qualitative methods to study subjective experience. This means listening to consumers and their families through first-person reports, essays, poetry, paintings, and commentaries, as well as attending informational sessions conducted by the individuals themselves (cf. Brekke *et al.*, 1993). The upsurge of interest among social scientists in qualitative methods is no doubt due in part to a growing recognition of the importance of phenomenology for a more complete understanding of human experience and behaviour.

THE TRANSACTIONAL MODEL

If we accept that the behaviour of people with disabilities is manifested in some environmental milieu with its unique opportunities and constraints, the outward performance of the individual should be viewed as an outcome of the person-interaction. Evans has pointed out that dispositional traits such as self-esteem, locus of control and hardiness

will interact with environmental events and vicissitudes to determine
the resultant level of QOL. High self-esteem, internal locus of control,
and hardiness can mitigate the effects of negative events so that QOL
remains unscathed. However, very prolonged environmental stress
and continual disappointments could, in the absence of social support,
eventually have a detrimental effect on personality itself such that all
self-confidence and resilience are destroyed.

We recognize that the relative strengths of the personal versus environmental determinants of an individual's performance may vary from
person to person. In any case, it does seem that to the extent to which
the behaviour of the individual can be enhanced, hinges partly on inner
resources, the perception of barriers, and the contingencies of the external environment. The person-environment transactional model would
suggest that these factors are components of a total interacting system (Lawton, 1983). The environmental factors, according to Lawton
(1983), may take many forms; for example, low income, poor health, a
lack of accessible age-relevant opportunities, a shrinking of the available
social network, and environmental barriers such as poor transportation
and neighbourhood, which may all conspire to lowering the perceived
and achieved QOL of all individuals.

The growing recognition of the multiplicity of factors that affect
an individual's QOL perceptions and evaluations is reflected in the
widespread adoption of "systems paradigms." According to this approach, the individual profile of QOL is best conceptualized in terms
of a number of different levels – psychological, ecological, cultural
– which may influence one another. Consequently, we have to consider the *interdependence* of these levels, and the dynamic interaction
of demands and responses of the QOL expectations associated with
them.

ENVIRONMENTAL OPPORTUNITIES

To bring about an improvement in QOL, it may be easier to modify
environments than to change people (cf. Feather, 1990). Positive
perceptions of QOL are likely to be fostered by environments that permit

the satisfaction of using new and old skills. It frequently happens among the disabled population that they are not allowed to practice their skills. Thus, elderly people may be forced to retire from their jobs because of their age or infirmity, those with chronic physical illnesses may have to quit prematurely because they can no longer cope, mentally disordered individuals may be dismissed because they are incompetent or difficult to work with, and those with developmentally disabilities may not even find meaningful work in the first place because they are never given a chance. The importance of employment for keeping occupied and satisfying both material needs and personal dignity cannot be overestimated. However, work environments that pressure people to comply with the demands of others tend to cause distress. Conversely, being able to generate one's own goals and pattern them after one's own values and beliefs is conducive to a better QOL.

There is general agreement that personal autonomy is a major ingredient of QOL. The empowerment of consumers of long-term care, and their families, is both an end in itself and a means of enhancing QOL. Nevertheless, there is considerable variability in individual preferences for autonomy. Certain individuals may prefer the comfort and security of an institution to having to fend for themselves in the community. And sometimes a conflict exists between mental health workers eager to have their clients living in the community and the parents of these clients who would prefer to see them looked after in an institution. From a QOL standpoint, it is for the individuals themselves to choose and decide on the degree of independence they feel comfortable with.

Related to the concept of autonomy is the concept of control. Opportunity for controlling and modifying environmental contingencies promotes feelings of self-efficacy and self-worth which in turn, consistent with top-down theories of QOL, lead to greater life satisfaction (Rodin, 1989). But although the opportunity for control usually leads to positive outcomes in terms of QOL, there are exceptions. Rodin *et al.* (1980) point out that some individuals who are disabled may not wish to exercise control, and shun the responsibility, because they are worried that the decisions they take may not turn out to be in their best interests. For instance, a person suffering from schizophrenia or agoraphobia who is afraid of facing the world outside may choose to spend all day at home in bed. Even though this lifestyle may have suited Goncharov's character Oblomov, it is clearly maladaptive behaviour.

So far we have been assuming, of course, that we are able to exercise some degree of control over our environment. But what of those environments that promote opportunity for control over events that are actually uncontrollable? Attempts to attain control over these events could elicit a high investment of time and effort that are intrinsically futile. Furthermore, as Ory and Cox have indicated, "individual preferences for control differ widely and variability for preferred levels of control may increase with age." Nevertheless, for most people the perceived power to control events (internal locus of control) is an asset and is associated with a higher QOL. This is why living in institutional settings, where there is a greater risk of losing perceived control and autonomy, is considered less desirable from the point of view of QOL than living in the community.

The phrase "variety is the spice of life" takes on new meaning for people with disabilities. Interventions to prevent boredom, morbidity and passivity resulting from being unable to participate in age-compatible activities are needed to promote QOL. To be successful such interventions should require both physical and intellectual activities. On the other hand, *novelty* has its drawbacks for people who like to be able to forecast what is probably going to happen to them in the future. There needs to be a balance between novelty, to prevent boredom, etc., and continuity, to prevent uncertainty. Where this balance should lie will depend on the population, e.g., young versus old, and ultimately on the individual within that population.

Bringing together results of studies conducted within the theoretical framework proposed by Altman and Chemers (1987), it can tentatively be concluded that environments of those who are frail and elderly, physically disabled, and mentally challenged which demand very close interpersonal contact and do not allow for personal boundaries, are likely to have negative effects upon their mental health and QOL. At the same time, restricted opportunities for interpersonal contacts are expected to have similar negative effects. In determining a social environment that maximizes QOL for all individuals, young and old, it must be designed such that it allows sufficient privacy but precludes isolation, and encourages interaction but avoids high density, since excesses in both directions can be psychologically harmful.

MODERN TECHNOLOGY

Czaja and Barr (1989) observe that a coincidence of two trends – the current technological revolution, and the rapid increase in the size of the older population and the number of individuals with special need for rehabilitation – has created an urgent need to consider the characteristics, capacities, and limitations of individuals who are disabled and frail in relation to new technologies. Everyday encounters and interactions with technology have made increasing numbers of adults who are old and frail, and others with physically disabilities living in the general population more determined to seek a better quality of life by becoming more aggressive and active users of the assistive technologies, rather than be just passive recipients of technological aids that are designed for general consumers.

The dilemma we face as a society is that social and medical ethics oblige manufacturers, physicians, and researchers to promote new technologies in an effort to postpone the individual's dependence on others. Autonomy, self-management, and self-reliance are constructs vitally tied in with the self-esteem of all individuals, both young and old. The emergence of a technological revolution has occurred at a time when the average number of years that people spend physically disabled, sensorily impaired, or mobility impaired has grown faster than those they spend healthily. In other words, although people are enjoying more healthy years while they are young and middle-aged, they may be paying the price for a higher QOL by spending more time disabled when they are older (Olshansky et al., 1993).

Data already indicate that more and more older adults already feel the pressure to learn to use computers and other new technologies in order to maintain some respectability in their QOL, and in their personal and recreational pursuits. For manufacturers and service providers, it is becoming increasingly apparent that designing technologies for an assumed-to-be homogeneous population is unnecessarily limiting.

Instead, technological change must take into account the whole range of physical, sensory, and cognitive abilities, skills and impairments that exist in among the full population. Failure on the part of educators, sociologists, manufacturers of technology, and consumers to consider this diversity both limits the usefulness of innovative assistive technologies, and creates an increasingly large group of older adults and disabled youth frustrated by the very technological change that should have improved their QOL (Stagner, 1985).

In the not too distant future there will be programmable wheelchairs, voice-activated computer control centres, and robots that aid in the performance of tasks such as meal preparation, and the like. Ways must be found to make the cost of such equipment within the reach of the intended users. The obvious task is to convince the private and public sector that this type of equipment is effective in maintaining independence, both physical and psychological, and will help to enrich the QOL of those in need.

If brand new products, modifications to existing products, services for clients, and advice to consumers concerning assistive tools are to be successful, consideration of these products needs to be given greater priority. Effective research on assistive technology from the consumers' viewpoint requires that information be drawn from "focus groups" rather than from general volunteers. For example, focus groups consisting of experts in mobility impairment, sensory impairment, and cognitive impairment should be used to identify and prioritize factors that consumers use to evaluate devices. A number of gerontologists, especially Nagi (1990) and Strain *et al.* (1993), have proposed the formation of legalized partnership between governmental agencies, researchers, manufacturers, retailers, service providers, and consumers of all ages. This would entail matching the needs and interests of all partners. Because the types of technical information frequently requested by manufacturers, retailers and service providers often pose considerable difficulties for the consumers, all partnerships must involve the participation of ombudsmen and well informed caregivers who have the time to observe the actual functioning of disabled individuals using the assistive technologies. In addition, confidentiality must be respected if manufacturers are going to be given access to potential users of their products.

In many ways the QOL issue is a difficult one. Although it is often portrayed in health studies as being associated with critical intervention and the right to treatment, QOL is in fact associated with a wide range of daily activities, many of which are insignificant when taken separately, but are important to QOL when taken cumulatively. Individuals who learn to cope better in later life may do so because they have learnt to cope over a lifetime. This accentuates the incremental nature of QOL and the importance of focusing of QOL throughout life rather than at any particular point in time. Yet QOL studies seem to have had relatively little influence on education, including special education. Although it can be argued that many of the issues concerning education involve QOL, such as resource enrichment, professional education, changes to the design of schools, or individual educational planning, few articles actually state QOL as their major focus (see Timmons, 1993).

Barton (1992) notes that the examination of official and academic records clearly shows the absence of the views of people who are disabled. This he indicates is particularly relevant in the field of education where it is suggested that few studies voicing the consumers' concerns exist. Children probably represent the least empowered of citizens. Their voice is heard through those representing them, generally parents, and to some extent, lawyers and health professionals, but these are the very groups that researchers, working in the QOL field for adults, have concerns about. Advocacy is seen as extremely important, and has eloquently been described in various forms by Neufeld (1991), who argues that quality services in special needs areas have relevance to all children. Self-advocacy has possibilities, but in the area of education the opinions of children are not often sought. Indeed it is the deliberate involvement of the child in developmental strategies and problem solving which would come to the fore in QOL studies undertaken on children.

Within special education the production of individual educational plans, that are required at least in the US, provides some opportunity for child input. However, an examination of teenagers' perceptions indicates that children with disabilities are much more controlled than children without disabilities (Brown and Timmons, 1993). This control results from environmental situations, and teacher and parent behaviour. For instance, bedtimes of children who are disabled are controlled by parents but self-monitored by similarly aged children who do not have disabilities. Again, children in special classes often eat meals alone unlike children without disabilities, and friendships are severely controlled and limited. Inspection of Halpern's list of QOL domains reveals that some of them appear to be transgressed in these examples (i.e., personal relations and social networks are being restricted).

Day Care in Canada (Johnson and Dineer, 1981) is seen as being in a state of crisis with conditions that raise major concerns about the care and development of children. Yet, again, there is a dearth of studies which relate directly to QOL of very young children though there have been studies on topics which are connected. Our point is that unless there is a *holistic* consideration of child education, welfare and development in terms of an overriding and comprehensive model, research and policy will continue to be conducted on a piecemeal basis. The advantage of a QOL framework is that it provides a structure for longitudinal studies which consider the child (and adult) from multiple perspectives, including the perceptions of the individuals themselves.

LOBBYING AND POLICY MAKING

A number of developments over the past decade have been associated with empowerment and choice, quite separately from research into QOL. The development of associations of people with disabilities, the organization of other consumer groups and the growth of these into national and international bodies is a reflection of greater empowerment amongst the population. As a consequence, joint workshops and conferences between consumers and professionals have become more common, e.g., the Canadian Down Syndrome Association and the

National Down Syndrome Association in the US. Of course, in these latter instances, it is generally the parents who advocate on behalf of their children.

In the health field, the recent first Canadian forum on breast cancer (November, 1993) included women who had been treated for breast cancer. They made up 25% of the delegates and had a major impact on program content. Such lobbying is affecting government policy, but also helps to empower individuals who wish to access services.

The development of personal support groups, such as the Joshua committees (Marlett *et al.*, 1984), illustrate how group organization over individual cases can change funding strategies. Individualized funding, which attaches dollars to the individual or his/her family, is now becoming recognized in North America in the field of disability. With legislation and financial resources, empowerment and choice are moved away from professional domination to the consumer and, with a more equal share of the power, the involvement of the consumer in decision making. Individuals being responsible for their own health becomes a real possibility. In turn, such developments lead to the practice of brokerage where individuals can be assisted to find the professional services they feel best meet their needs. However, this assumes the availability of services from which to make a choice. There are also other issues that have yet to be resolved.

Many professionals do not feel that individual consumers are informed enough to make meaningful choices, and government may question whether individuals will use funding appropriately. Although these issues have to a large degree evolved separately from the research field of QOL, similar trends are apparent. They both represent the greater involvement of the individual in selection, deployment of resources and evaluation of service delivery. The research on QOL provides tools through which knowledge, opinions and choices can be better utilized by the consumer. It suggests that professionals must come to view their clients and the method by which the service is delivered in a new light. These changes are well documented in the current set of papers, and are to some degree exemplified by the current consumer movements. It seems likely that the coming decade will not only feature QOL studies in increasing volume but will also see major changes in the perceptions of all parties, and this will dramatically reshape both research and practice.

With respect to social policy on financing superior QOL for all individuals, both typical and atypical, what is required and desirable is a close partnership of the private and public sectors than can bring about a creative mix of voluntary inputs from community, private initiatives in preventive medicine, and new programs of public entitlement that encourage the participation of all individuals in active and healthy lifestyles. What is needed then is some sort of balance between the medical and the social types of intervention.

Not only do consumers but also researchers need to lobby in order to get their research results across. There needs to be closer consultation among researchers and policy makers. Ory and Cox make the point that "any success towards improving the quality of life for groups of older people will be limited if the information is not effectively communicated or deemed as relevant by practitioners, program administrators or policy makers." (This is true of course for other groups besides those who are elderly.) Ory and Cox then go on to make a number of useful recommendations for achieving this end.

ACTIVE CITIZENSHIP

Provision of appropriate environmental opportunities for individuals with disabilities, who are often unable to speak up for themselves, is a task that has been shouldered by consumer advocates. That we also, as focal groups of concerned citizens in Western societies, position ourselves as advocates and gatekeepers for the QOL of the population at large in the midst of our rapidly changing society is crucial. We have a responsibility to modify semi-pathological environments that mitigate against improving QOL and to assist our communities as they adjust to changes that are often beyond the personal control of individuals who are frail, disabled and frequently depressed. It is worth remembering that although our short-term and long-term concern with identifying QOL indicators (whether objective or subjective) should be pursued for reasons of immediate relevance to public policy or to any particular group of disadvantaged individuals, this objective is not sufficient. We, as responsible citizens, should be equally motivated to contribute to a more generalized enlightenment of humane society concerned with self-evaluation and the improvement of QOL for all individuals at various stages of personal and social development, and with all individuals showing substantial departures from the norm in their economic, social, and ecological status which adversely affect their QOL.

REFERENCES

Andrews, F. M. and S. B. Withey: 1976, Social Indicators of Well Being: Americans' Perceptions of Life Quality (Plenum, New York).

Autio, T.: 1992, The Quality of Life of Mentally Retarded: Interviewing Results in Tabular Form (Finnish Association of Mental Retardation Research and Experimental Unit, Helsinki).

Barton, L.: 1992, 'Disability and the necessity for a socio-political perspective', in L. Barton, K. Ballard and G. Fulcher (eds.), Disability and the Necessity for a Socio-Political Perspective, Monograph No. 51 (The International Exchange of Experts and Information in Rehabilitation, University of New Hampshire, Durham, NH).

Bateson, G.: 1972, Steps to an Ecology of Mind (Chandlerpun, San Francisco).

Berkman, L. F. and L. B. Breslow: 1989, Health and Ways of Living: The Alameda County Study (Oxford University Press, Oxford).

Borgen, W. and N. Amundson: 1984, The Experience of Unemployment: Implications for Counselling the Unemployed (Nelson, Scarborough, ON).

Brekke, J. S., S. Levin, G. H. Wolkon and E. Slade: 1993, 'Psychosocial functioning and subjective experience in schizophrenia', Schizophrenia Bulletin 19, pp. 599–608.

Brown, R. I.: 1992, 'Aging and the arts', in R. I. Brown, H. Coward and J. Dugan (eds.), Arts: The Soul of the Community (Institute for the Humanities, Calgary).

Brown, R. I., M. B. Bayer and C. MacFarlane: 1989, Rehabilitation Programmes: Performance and Quality of Life of Adults with Developmental Handicaps (Lugus, Toronto).

Brown, R. I., M. B. Bayer and P. M. Brown: 1992, Empowerment and Developmental Handicaps: Choices and Quality of Life (Captus University Publications, Toronto; Chapman and Hall, London).

Brown, R. I. and V. Timmons: 1993, 'Quality of Life – Adults and adolescents with disabilities', Forthcoming in Exceptionality Education in Canada.

Bruhn, J. G. and B. U. Philips: 1984, 'Measuring social support: A synthesis of current approaches', Journal of Behavioral Medicine 7, pp. 151–169.

Calman, K. C.: 1984, 'Quality of life in cancer patients – An hypothesis', Journal of Medical Ethics 10, pp. 124–127.

Campbell, A.: 1983, The Sense of Well-Being in America (McGraw-Hill, New York).

Clark, P. G.: 1988, 'Autonomy, personal empowerment, and quality of life in long-term care', Journal of Applied Gerontology 7, pp. 179–194.

Cummins, R. A.: 1992, Comprehensive Quality of Life Scale – Intellectual Disability ComQol-ID Manual 3rd ed. (Deakin University, Toorak, Australia).

Czaja, S. J. and R. A. Barr: 1989, 'Technology and the everyday life of older adults', Annals of the American Academy of Political and Social Science 503, pp. 127–137.

Day, H. I.: 1989, 'Quality of life of people with disabilities', Keynote Address, 4th Canadian Congress of Rehabilitation, Toronto.

Denholm, C. J.: 1993, 'Developmental needs of adolescents; application to adolescents with Down Syndrome', in R. I. Brown (ed.), Building our Future (Proceedings of the 1992 National Conference of the Canadian Down's Syndrome Society, Rehabilitation Studies, University of Calgary, Calgary).

Edgerton, R.: 1990, 'Quality of life from a longitudinal research perspective', in R. Schalock and M. Begab (eds.), Quality of Life: Perspectives and Issues (American Association on Mental Retardation, Washington, DC).

Emes, C. and B. Ferris: 1986, Physical Activities Amongst Activity-limited and Disabled Canadians (Fitness Canada, Ottawa).

Erickson, E. H.: 1968, Identity, Youth and Crisis (Norton, New York).

Feather, N. T. (ed.): 1980, Expectancy, Incentive, and Action (Erlbaum, Hillsdale, NJ).

Felce, D. and J. Perry: 1993, 'Quality of life: A contribution to its definition and measurement'. Unpublished report, Mental Handicap in Wales Applied Resource Unit, Cardiff.

Felton, B. J. and T. A. Revenson: 1987, Age differences in coping with chronic illness', Psychology and Aging 2, pp. 164–170.

Firth, H. and M. Rapley: 1990, From Acquaintance to Friendship: Issues for People with Learning Disabilities (BIMH Publications, Kidderminster).

Halpern, A. S., G. Nave, D. W. Close and D. Nelson: 1986, 'An empirical analysis of the dimensions of community adjustment for adults with mental retardation', Australia and New Zealand Journal of Developmental Disabilities 12, pp. 147–157.

Hofstede, G.: 1984, 'The cultural relativity of the quality of life concept', Academy of Management Review 9, pp. 389–398.

Johnson, L. C. and J. Dineer: 1982, The Kin Trade: The Day Care Crisis in Canada (McGraw-Hill Ryerson, Toronto).

Lance, C. E., G. L. Lautenschlager, C. E. Sloan and P. E. Varca: 1989, 'A comparison between bottom-up, top-down, and bidirectional models of relationships between global and life facet satisfaction', Journal of Personality 57, pp. 601–624.

Lawton, M. P.: 1983, 'The varieties of well-being', Experimental Aging Research 9, pp. 65–72.

Lehman, A. F.: 1983, 'The well-being of chronic mental patients: Assessing their quality of life', Archives of General Psychiatry 40, pp. 369–373.

Marcia, J. E.: 1966, 'Development and validation of ego-identify status', Journal of Personality and Social Psychology 3, pp. 551–558.

Marlett, N. J., R. Gall and A. Wight-Felske: 1984, Dialogue on Disability: A Canadian Perspective (University of Calgary Press, Calgary).

Maslow, A. H.: 1968, Toward a Psychology of Being 2nd ed. (Van Nostrand Rheinhold, New York).

McIntyre, K., M. Farrell and A. David: 1989, 'In-patient psychiatric care: The patient's view', British Journal of Medical Psychology 62, pp. 249–255.

Mercier, C. and S. King: in press, 'A latent variable causal model of the quality of life and community tenure of psychotic patients', Forthcoming in American Journal of Psychiatry.

Nagi, S. Z.: 1990, 'Disability concepts revisited: Implications for prevention. Appendix A', in A. M. Pope and A. R. Tarlov (eds.), Disability in America: A National Agenda for Prevention (National Academy Press, Washington, DC), pp. 216–227.

Neufeld, R.: 1991, 'Advocacy: Applications in early years of children', in D. Mitchell and R. I. Brown (eds.), Early Intervention: Studies for Young Children with Special Needs (Chapman and Hall, London).

Olshansky, S. J., B. A. Carnes and C. K. Cassel: 1993, 'The aging of the human species', Scientific American, April, pp. 46–52.

Osaba, D.: 1991, Effect of Cancer on Quality of Life (CRC Press, Baca Raton, FL).

Pinkney, A. A., G. J. Gerber and H. G. Lafave: 1991, 'Quality of life after psychiatric rehabilitation: The clients' perspective', Acta Scandinavica Psychiatrica 83, pp. 86–91.

Rodin, J.: 1989, 'Sense of control: Potentials for intervention', Annals of the American Academy of Political and Social Science 503, pp. 29–42.

Rodin, J., K. Rennert and S. K. Solomon: 1980, 'Intrinsic motivation for control: Fact or fiction', in A. Baum and J. E. Singer (eds.), Advances in Environmental Psychology, Vol. 2 (Erlbaum, Hillsdale, NJ), pp. 131–148.

Romney, D. M.: 1994, 'Psychosocial functioning and subjective experience in schizophrenia: A reanalysis using LISREL', Paper submitted for publication.

Romney, D. M., C. D. Jenkins and J. M. Bynner: 1992, 'A structural analysis of health-related quality of life dimensions', Human Relations 45, pp. 165–176.

Rotter, J. B.: 1966, 'Generalized expectancies for internal versus external locus of control', Psychological Monographs 80, pp. 1–28.

Rowland, J. H.: 1989, 'Developmental stage and adaptation: Adult model', in J. D. Holland and J. H. Rowland (eds.), Handbook of Psycho-oncology: Psychological Care of the Patient with Cancer (Oxford University Press, New York), pp. 25–43.

Sartorius, N: 1987, 'Cross-cultural comparisons of data about quality of life: A sample of issues', in N. K. Aaronson and J. Beckman (eds.), The Quality of Life of Cancer Patients (Raven, New York), pp. 19–24.

Schalock, R. L.: 1990, Quality of Life: Perspectives and Issues (American Association on Mental Retardation, Washington, DC).

Schalock, R. L.: 1991, 'The concept of quality of life in the lives of persons with mental retardation', Paper presented at the 115th Annual Meeting of the American Association on Mental Retardation, Washington, DC.

Schipper, H., J. Clinch, A. McMurray and M. Levitt: 1984, 'Measuring the quality of life of cancer patients: Development and validation', Journal of Clinical Oncology 2, pp. 472–483.

Shotton, M. A.: 1985, 'Belt up – if you can', Applied Ergonomics 11, pp. 127-133.

Stagner, R.: 1985, 'Aging in industry', in J. E. Birren and K. W. Schaie (eds.), Handbook of the Psychology of Aging 2nd ed. (Van Nostrand Reinhold, New York).

Stokols, D.: 1992, 'Establishing and maintaining health environments: Towards a social ecology of health promotion', American Psychologist 47, pp. 6–22.

Strain, L. A., N. L. Chappell and M. J. Penning: 1993, 'The need for social science research on technology and aging', Technology and Disability 2, pp. 56–64.

Thapa, K. and L. A. Rowland: 1989, 'Quality of life perspectives in long-term care: Staff and patient perceptions', Acta Psychiatrica Scandinavica 80, pp. 267–271.

Timmons, T.: 1993, Quality of Life of Teenagers with Special Needs (Doctoral dissertation, University of Calgary).

Warr, P.: 1987, Work, Unemployment and Mental Health (Clarendon Press, Oxford).

WHO: 1980, International Classification of Impairments, Disabilities and Handicaps (World Health Organization, Geneva).

Wolfensberger, W.: 1983, 'Social role valorization: A proposed new term for the principle of normalization', Mental Retardation 21, pp. 234–239.

Zautra, A. J. and J. W. Reich: 1983, 'Life events and perceptions of quality of life: Developments in a two factor approach', Journal of Community Psychology 11, pp. 121–132.

The University of Calgary,
Faculty of Education,
Dept. of Education Psychology,
Calgary, Alberta,
Canada.